OX-BOW

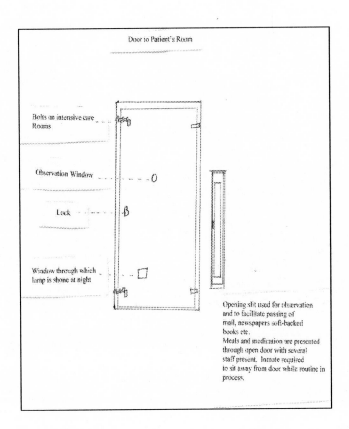

Door to Patient's Room

Bolts on intensive care Rooms

Observation Window

Lock

Window through which lamp is shone at night

Opening slit used for observation and to facilitate passing of mail, newspapers soft-backed books etc.
Meals and medication are presented through open door with several staff present. Inmate required to sit away from door while routine in process.

By Janet Cresswell

Published by:
Chipmunkapublishing
PO Box 6872
Brentwood
Essex
CM13 1ZT
United Kingdom

http://www.chipmunkapublishing.com

ISBN   978 1 84747 017 1

The development of this book was made possible by a grant from The Arts Council, London.

The Concise Oxford Dictionary definition of ox-bow: A loop formed by a horseshoe bend in a river.

CONTENTS

FOREWORD

Janet Cresswell tells all in this amazingly revealing autobiography. Janet lived in Broadmoor hospital for over 25 years. She writes with great honsety, integrity and bravery. The circumstances to which Janet Creswell became a mental health patient are completely unfair. Creswell reveals in her own words how she became a victim of the British Medical Profession and psychiatry. The fact that this story has not been heard in full by the general public is a travesty. In 2003 Janet Creswell was released from Broadmoor and remains in a secure hospital unit today. Creswell writes in detail of her growing up during the war. Married with a child and working for a living all seemed normal until doctors intervened and ruined her life. Creswell reveals what living in Broadmoor has really been like, the mindset and behaviour of the nurses and psychiatrists and her relationships with other patients. The publication of this books marks a period in history where mental health patients are getting their voices heard. It is impossible to stop the voice of the mental health patients around the world as we move onwards and upwards in the 21st Century. Janet Creswell should be applauded for having the bravery to write this memoir.

Jason Pegler CEO of Chipmunkapublishing

INTRODUCTION- FOUNDING OF AN EMPIRE

Those swept into the mental health empire frequently have no understanding of what besets them and I have been no different. Although I kept a diary all I have now relates to a few months at the end of 1990 into 1991 from which this book evolves with flashes both forward and backwards. I spent a quarter of a century at Broadmoor and for those, like I was once – unaware of what the place is about – I include this glimpse at its history and the beginnings of the empire of which Broadmoor is a small part.

It was in the reign of Henry VIII when a kindly judge realised that the prisoner in the dock had no knowledge of the murder for which he was accused and spared the man being sent to the gallows; he decreed the man was insane and should be sent to a mental institution. Whether the prisoner was insane or innocent history does not record but this method of so evading the death penalty, with most pleading epilepsy, impossible to disprove until the advent of electroencephalogram (EEG) machines, became practice within the penal system. That it was irrational to hang the sane and preserve the insane was never an issue nor was the impossibility of diagnosing sanity or insanity. It can be assumed, however, that those with sufficient funds to employ top legal advisers were those committed and stayed alive whilst the poor hung. It may well be that the financial status of those originally detained at Broadmoor influenced the allowed budget which was always far higher than allotted for the prisons.

The overcrowding both in prisons and mental institutions was also a criteria in deciding a verdict; both Timothy Evans, wrongfully charged for a 10 Rillington Place murder, and Ruth Ellis who shot her lover outside the *Magdala* public house in Hampstead, should both have been sent to either Rampton or Broadmoor, Evans because he was sub-normal and Ellis because hers was *crime passionale* which in another country would have exonerated her. Both hung. It was only the insistence of the distraught parents of Timothy Evans, with the help of their MP that got the case re-opened and the slowness of the Home Office to admit an innocent man had hanged caused a public uproar. Thus the Mental Health Act (MHA) was founded on fraud although originally and sometimes for humanitarian purposes.

The protests at Evans' death made it inevitable from the early 1950's that capital punishment would be abolished (1964) which meant that psychiatrists would no longer be required in court to advise on mental state. This situation was avoided by a flood of publicity on new treatments and, showing great boldness, the MHA 1959 allowed for a far wider range of admittances than previously covered. There was no allowance for those wrongly committed, no admission of bad clinical judgement, and the frequent grievous results of forced treatments of which LSD (lysergic acid diethylamide) was one and withdrawn only after pressure from newspapers. It is under this Act that I was swept into a maelstrom from which I have struggled for understanding and release. At the time there was a massive rise in prison transfers, committals via social workers and the Police, much of which could be termed over-zealous "dumping", and ease of management, regardless of the result. This increase of tempo and lack of redress triggered the start of the User – to become Refuser – Movement that protested at the 'weapons' of psychiatry. One of the first was Mental Patients Union situated in a squat house in Hackney, which produced a leaflet detailing the side effects of psychiatric medication. The idea behind this was to have this medication withdrawn or curtailed but it was the drug manufacturers who were the main purchasers of the leaflet and it is now standard practice to include a list of side effects as though these effects are acceptable. The 1983 MHA endeavoured to provide protection for users with the formation of the Mental Health Commissioners - made up of members of the psychiatric profession who were given no elbow to enforce justice where necessary - and more Mental Health Tribunals with a psychiatrist on the panel with a brief to examine 'fitness to leave', 'wrongful committal' was not catered for and Appeals Courts maintained that those committed under the Mental Health Act could be heard by Mental Health Tribunals. Thus the system flourished with enormously inflated administration costs and no satisfaction to the claimant.

Over the years law makers have indulged in academic nuances such as changing committals from "Not guilty by reason of insanity", to "Guilty but insane" and back again; "sub-normality" to "impairment" and (on discharge) "satisfied that a patient is not suffering from a disorder" to "not satisfied that a patient is suffering from a disorder". The basic issue that there are no means of assessing sanity or insanity, even with the 1959 and 1983 (Amendment) Acts, has never been mentioned. The Angela Canning verdict (2004) on cot deaths, which decreed that a person should not be convicted on "opinion" should alter the thinking behind the proposed changes of the Act under review and it is to be hoped that a get-out such as "a prisoner is **convicted** and a patient **committed**, thus a patient can be put away on opinion" is not adopted. As it is, the fraud perpetuated in the 16th Century continues into the 21st.

In 1700 the population of the UK was four and a half million, rising to twenty million in 1800, causing widespread housing shortage, unemployment, poverty and crime. The prisons were overflowing and, when America gained Independence in 1776 and refused to accept more felons for its convict colonies, from this country, it was publicly announced that, as a great social experiment, Australia would be used as a penal settlement.

The first transportation was hailed as a historic event and a great deal written about it at the time but, although not publicly advertised, most historians agree that the colony was started to conceal the trading posts set up in Australia for business with the Orient. In plain words, the transportation of prisoners to relieve over-crowded prisons in the UK, caused by population expansion, was a cover for the opium trade.

The policy of transporting prisoners, many of whom had committed very minor offences, was regarded by many as a means to cover gross corruption considered necessary by some for the economy of the country as much as to ease over-crowding. It came to an end in 1863. During the previous eighty years, forty of them containing great protest, 161,000 prisoners were transported, one third of them Irish; the barbaric fashion was terminated, not so much on humanitarian grounds, but mainly from complaint by some Australian land owners that they had not been allowed what they considered to be their fair share of cheap labour. It says something for the weight of 19thC protestors that other overseas British penal colonies were not created in India or Africa.The French also enjoyed a similar practice, with its use of Devil's Island off the coast of Cayenne, Guiana, which was not abolished until 1945.

The termination of transportation brought great strain to bear on the British government who were unused to dealing with its penal system in any other terms than rough justice and removing offenders out of sight. Transportation was a far more imposing term than dumping and removal of social dissidents a far simpler solution than addressing the problems represented many of them emanating from the housing and employment situation. A massive building programme was introduced and many of the UK's existing prisons and mental hospitals, including Broadmoor, were built at that time, in the mid 19th century, mainly in the remote open countryside that today is valuable building land. To take the overflow from Bethlem Lunatic Asylum, Broadmoor was built in 1863, designed by Sir Joshua Webb. It was completed in two years with prison labour making the best of southern aspect with beautiful views across the Berkshire countryside and sunny high- ceiling rooms; it was typical of other mental asylums constructed across the UK over the same period and reflected a compassionate attitude to those incarcerated within the walls. Like most, Broadmoor was self-supporting as far as possible with its own farm and extensive vegetable gardens and orchard. It grew large patches of rhubarb, a considered cure for insanity of the age.

Compare this with the new building project of the 1980's sited in a hollow; it took ten years with outside contractors, was over £30K overspent on the first phase and required the help of disc jockey, Sir Jimmy Savile, to complete.

The advent of new treatments, electro-convulsive therapy (ECT) and medication, made psychiatrists keen to extend their practise outside the usual epileptic/subnormal/murderer so pressure was exerted to introduce the 1948 MHA which allowed voluntary patients to be admitted to hospital. It was the 1959 MHA, however, which sought to recognise psychiatric treatment as curative and thus give credence to release from Broadmoor, often through the general mental hospital system which made law the concept of indefinite detention until cured. That this is an ideal and not a pragmatic approach to affecting a flow of patients in and out of special hospital has never been acknowledged. There is no means of testing for insanity or sanity and therefore a cure is difficult if not impossible to prove scientifically; trying to prove either condition can cause undue stress to patients who are frequently pressurised to agree to treatments that are cures in name only but look good on paper. The 1959 Act widened the scope of those committed and Broadmoor changed its name from Criminal Lunatic Asylum to Special Hospital, its crockery ceased to be stamped BCLA and male staff uniforms bore the new logo.

Despite optimism on the subject, the flow rate remained slow and ground to a standstill in the late 70's when members of the Confederation of Health Service Employees (COHSE) went on strike in protest at Broadmoor patients being transferred to ordinary mental hospitals. There has always been a strange reluctance to impose definite sentences that would remove the necessity for subterfuge to affect release and it must be supposed that the claim that this is in the interests of the public has some substance. It would be churlish to suppose that the lawyers and consultants who comprise the bodies of experts to assess release aspects would face unemployment if the system were abolished or amended to more reasonable proportions.

Over the years alterations to laws pertaining to the penal system have been forced on successive governments of all parties, in most cases these legal amendments have related to lack of integrity in some members of authority. For instance, the Capital Punishment Amendment Act (1868) was introduced preventing discharge of the death penalty for three weeks after sentence had been pronounced as a prisoner had been hanged before the evidence proving his innocence was available. The law was again amended to ensure the transfer of prisoners from remand to place of destination three weeks after sentencing and the reason for this is not hard to determine. There has been prison overcrowding for at least two centuries and it is not difficult to imagine the protests of Prison Governors and their staff at news of more arrivals if those already housed have long sentences still to serve. It was only riots in the 1990's at Strangeways, Wakefield and so on that produced a review of the conditions in which prisoners are held.

When the wrongful hanging of Timothy Evans came to light in the early 1950's the public outcry was so great that the Government was forced to reconsider the death penalty which was repealed in 1964. That the

Home Office was so slow to admit the miscarriage of justice and to the end protested that Evans had murdered his child in anguish at finding his wife dead, brought home to many the reluctance of those in authority to admit what in others would be termed a reprehensible cover-up for an error of judgement. This refusal to accept responsibility for such error is regarded as a symptom of schizophrenia in those labelled mentally ill and sufficient grounds to refuse parole in a convicted prisoner; it is obvious that, throughout its history, those in control of the penal system have not addressed the main issues and have allowed themselves variants in behaviour that is condemned in those committed or convicted. Equally the practice of exaggerating the prisoner's crimes to secure a committal is a symptom of paranoia. The Access to Medical Records Act (1987) made it possible to those committed to see what was written about them and understand that, in many instances, their misdeeds had been enlarged, before that time they were given no inkling of how their records depicted them.

Privately Home Office personnel admitted that, in 1973, they felt a third of all convicted prisoners were innocent, and so psychiatrists who conducted a vigorous campaign to convince the public that there had been breakthroughs in treatment for mental illness, were gradually introduced in the prisons with a view to reducing the number of cases of injustice. The resulting paperwork and stress involved by those practising an inexact science is considered by many to far exceed any benefit that may have occurred. The numbers in prison claiming innocence have increased. The hospital (psychiatric) F Wing at Brixton sustained seven suicides in 1989 rising to fifteen a year later. At any time with a thousand men on remand two thousand psychiatric reports could be in circulation. Even today there is no admittance that there are no means of diagnosing sanity or insanity – it is impossible to determine whether a person is suffering from voices in the head or merely maintaining that their crime has been produced by this factor – so experts in human behaviour can only complicate an already unwieldy penal system. The British may say that theirs is the best system of justice in the world but reality shows it to be adept at concealing injustice. The MHA under which those found criminally insane are detained is an Act to be manipulated; it is an anomaly and there is a weight of opinion that considers Special Hospitals should be abolished and greater care facilities introduced to the prison system. In the 1990's there were approximately two thousand people held in Special Hospitals at Rampton, Ashworth and Broadmoor with a further thousand elsewhere in RSUs, (Regional Secure Units), this figure was reduced to about twelve hundred but is again rising with building projects in process at several RSUs where charges to local health authorities per person range from £200K (£3650pw) - £400Kp.a. (Old age pensioner homes charge around £35Kp.a.). Prisons cost £27K p.a.

In fifteen years the Managers of Broadmoor changed five times becoming Special Hospital Service Authority and by 2001 the West London Hospital Trust, several of the name changes involving the same personnel (original DHS staff) located at different addresses with different letterheads with the same filing cabinets. Those committed through the courts are under the auspice of the Home Office, originally C3 Division now named The Mental Health Unit.

That psychiatrists have not fulfilled the terms of their brief and the authorities seem unable to deal adequately with the problem of injustice is shown by the length of time and amount of effort that has been required by such groups as the Guildford Four and others to prove innocence and obtain release from prison and the high number of three hundred and fifty two recommendations for reform made by the Royal Commission on Criminal Justice published in July 1993. The loophole of reprieve from hanging through plea of insanity was manipulated and used when convenient, the criteria being the over-crowded state of the prisons and special hospitals as much as the power of legal persuasion and wealth of plaintiff. It is understood that the death sentence was imposed more frequently than necessary and the requirements of the MHA misinterpreted where convenient because of overcrowding at Special Hospitals such as Broadmoor but this fact was never public knowledge. At all times the law must appear capable of coping with the wayward in its midst regardless of evidence to the contrary.

Prison overcrowding, and the size of the dole queue, is a motivating factor in sentencing, many courts are pleased to accept mental hospital recommendations in lieu of further straining prison facilities. The fashion of committing, rather than sentencing, stemmed from the 1959 MHA which allowed this to occur, it resulted in the UK becoming the country with the highest mental hospital and prison population per capita in Western Europe. Even so it is estimated that there are convictions for barely 3% of all crimes committed, most of these offenders giving themselves up to comprise the penal population. The offenders of the remaining 97% of unsolved crime remain free members of the community and this brings into question the over-long sentences and harsh treatment advocated by several Home Secretaries and governments who use the platform of crime rate to secure votes.

Until the COHSE action there was no consideration for those law-abiding people in mental institutions faced with the situation of being housed alongside and often classified with similar psychiatric labels to criminals. By definition a criminal has committed a crime and a mental patient has been victimised. In theory those sent to special hospitals should be victims who have retaliated or hit back at aggressors yet there is often very little difference between a person given a definite sentence and sent to prison and one given an indefinite sentence and sent to Broadmoor. Frequently there is no difference and it is interesting that the MHA is still used within the penal system.

On the other hand it is not uncommon for prisoners convicted by the courts to prison to serve a fixed sentence to be transferred to a special hospital to serve an indefinite one, therefore overruling the verdict of the court. Peter Sutcliffe, the Yorkshire Ripper, was sent to prison for the murder of thirteen women. He was found sane by judge and jury yet he is in Broadmoor. He was transferred from Parkhurst after sustaining injury from other prisoners. It is patently ludicrous to label Sutcliffe insane for being beaten up and causing the authorities problems with regard to his safety. His transfer to Broadmoor was merely convenient and substantiated the psychiatric reports that had been disputed by the court.

Ronny Kray (a London gangland killer) was also sentenced by the courts to life imprisonment in prison with his twin brother Reggy but was transferred to Broadmoor as "suffering from schizophrenia" despite there being a hospital wing in Parkhurst, prison hospital wings these days being mainly concerned with psychiatric rather than physical complaints. Interestingly it is claimed that when the Krays held sway in London's East End, old ladies were safe to walk the streets at night without fear of attack. One man was transferred to Broadmoor half way through a four-year prison sentence and he stayed there another thirty years.

Conditions in special hospitals are considered superior to those pertaining to prison, they cost considerably more, and so it is readily admitted that such a transfer can work in the prisoner's favour in some cases release can be facilitated. If Broadmoor, as widely believed, is a soft option to prison for those considered to be hard-luck cases, the publicity by staff for greater emoluments for working in high security, and the difficulties to secure release, is a paradox.

After widespread disturbances in both prisons and mental hospitals at the end of the Labour Government's tenure in 1979, which had sanctioned Broadmoor's ten-year re-building programme, and a reduction in numbers to ease the overcrowding, the Thatcher Government introduced amendments to the MHA in 1983. At the time it was understood that the Department of Health, who then managed special hospitals were in favour of abolishing the MHA whilst the Home Office were adamant for its retention. The same situation exists in 2004. Whilst John Major's Government's Criminal Justice Act received a U-turn because of public pressure by those affected by it, the MHA Amendments (1983) was regarded by many as cosmetic dressing and protests to it dismissed or ignored. Mental Health Act Commissioners to look at complaints, Second Opinion Doctors (SODs) to investigate validity of medication and more failed largely because there was no room to admit cases of poor clinical treatment and the shortage of suitable housing for those requiring care in the community.

The aim of the Act was to get the mental health system to function, i.e. to cure and release. It is an ideal that the guilty be committed for psychiatric treatment and released when cured but the reality is not possible; mental illness and sanity cannot be identified and there is no cure for this situation. With a regular routine most prisoners/patients straighten out within a few days, weeks or months and expensive treatments are not required, but the public obviously would not tolerate quick release of murderers or rapists, despite a lack of clarity why rape is considered to be a form of mental illness, and so a process must be adhered to. This includes an expensive tribunal system.

Until 1983 a tribunal consisted of a barrister (Chairman), a psychiatrist and a layperson (magistrate or social worker). The 1983 Act replaced the barrister with a judge, tribunals to be compulsory every three years with voluntary ones annually. Until 1994 legal aid was available only for those qualifying for it. As with normal litigation, those without funds qualify for legal representation and those with some private income frequently do not qualify for, nor can afford legal aid. The Tribunal had access to discretionary funds to award legal aid to those who did not qualify

21

for it but for whom the Tribunal wished legally represented and ultimately legal aid was offered to everyone for Mental Health Tribunals.

It has been known for tribunals to last a week; generally they are over in half a day with the plaintiff being present for maybe an hour. The idea was admirable in concept and designed to remove the event of people needlessly languishing in places like Broadmoor for forty years. The system can operate for some but for those with grudges real or imaginary against the medical profession, particularly psychiatry, or any other section of authority, the situation is hopeless. Appeals against wrong committals are usually rejected by the Appeal Judges on grounds that the case can be dealt with by a tribunal yet the brief of mental health tribunals permits examination only of fitness to leave, not investigation into matters of injustice. The MHA is a law that can be manipulated freely by those in control whilst subduing or ignoring protests.

When founded Broadmoor was self-supporting with its own farm laundry and so on but over the years this independence has been eroded to the benefit of wholesale suppliers. After Straffen absconded from the farm and assaulted a child, the farm was let privately. The laundry is now dealt with centrally with other hospitals in the area and the metalwork shop closed for some years to open up again within the kitchen garden area specialising in such items as flower baskets.   Due to the recession and the emphasis on security such area as the kitchen became barred to patients and outside labour employed. Whereas all the socks, for instance, were machine knitted by the men and finished in the female sewing room, by 1980 socks were bought in from outside. Although patients made a few of the issued dresses, outside seamstresses were employed in the sewing room, later to be moved apart due to intervention by the Prison Officers' Association that their presence did not conform to security regulations. Issued clothing, now much less than it used to be, is purchased from outside suppliers. By 1987 there were few occupational areas other than the kitchen gardens, where anything other than handiwork was performed. It is not surprising that costs have risen astronomically.

In 1976 it cost £93 per week to keep a patient in Broadmoor. By 1993 this figure had risen to nearly £1200 per week – over £60,000 p.a. – and by 1998 to over £120K p.a. for one patient which many view as excessive in light of result. During the years 1987 – 93 the administration staff increased more than five times from twenty to over a hundred, whilst the numbers of detainees were reduced from over 700 in 1976 to under 500 by 1993, all these years being beset by upheavals in the form of inflation, later deflation and outbreaks of unrest resulting in wage awards throughout the Civil Service.

In 1993, not the first time in its history, the UK embarked on an official policy of "community care". After centuries of ignoring or dumping its social outcasts it sought to treat within the community. The few disasters involving mental patients that have occurred have been presented unrealistically and the term "care in the community" has become another term for "legalised harassment". The proposals of the Royal Society for Psychiatry were rejected by the House of Commons in July 1993 as a violation of human rights and the politics played by those who wish to maintain control over others has included the reduction in the movement rate from places like Broadmoor until the situation is resolved. At the present time the female wings at both Ashworth and Broadmoor are to be closed but there is a shortage of places for the women to be transferred to, not because the women are unfit but largely because of the slowness of the system at creating places. A greater understanding of the mal effects of unwanted, often needless, psychiatric treatment has still to be addressed and the needs of those in positions of control to qualify their employment needs addressing.

If the monies expended on secure units and administration of a system that is propped up with bureaucracy could be spent on communities in the form of better housing, entertainment, home helps for those who need it etc. the quality of life in the country could be far better than it is likely to be with the implementation of yet another Mental Health Act designed like the Hutton Report to evade the main problems.

CHAPTER I - BROADMOOR

At the sound of the Fire Alarm

The wait to make a telephone call was interrupted by a piercing oscillating wail. Fire alarm. Down the corridor we struggled in a straggly line, the penetrating noise from the bell making us stuff our fingers in our ears. Two nurses stood at the top of the stairs into the garden, one with a clipboard ticking off our names as we trundled past, the other "counting". "It's Lizzy", says Sheila as we reach the stairwell, away from staff, "they wouldn't let her have a couple of Panadol"; the fire engine is obliged to respond to all calls and costs £1500 a visit. "Nobody knew where the alarm bell was when I came here and we didn't even have fire practice for three years", I mutter back. What was it staff said when I enquired about fire drill, "The staff know what to do". They might but with thirty-eight women who did not, what could the outcome be?

Into the garden's chill air we trailed, it had rained a lot during the day. I took old Margaret's arm as she stood dazed and two staff carried her friend Lily – the *News of the World* had featured them both as 'Fiends of Broadmoor'; at the time I was sitting between the two old ladies in the Sewing Room but doubted I was considered the rose amongst the thorns. "Oh it's terrible", Margaret cries, "I don't know what day it is". "Not surprising", I say, "one day's much like another, it's Wednesday 30 October 1990", I say and she repeats it adding, "You took an overdose once. What can I do? I can't take any more".

"I don't know" I say somewhat surprised at the turn of topic, "but I don't thank 'em for keeping me alive."

"Me neither", she says as she clutches my arm harder and lowers herself onto a garden bench. She is old for her seventy three years, her diabetes a problem, she is often dizzy and relies on her even older friend, Lily, to provide her with the sweets to which she is denied – these make her dizzier than ever. The newer, better treatment for diabetes enabling sufferers to eat sweets and cakes had not yet been discovered.   For Margaret the diet was limited in the extreme, a special dish being sent from the kitchen marked, "Diabetic". For us there was a choice but for Margaret it was take it or leave it although there were occasions we would envy her the chicken leg while we had macaroni or indeterminate stew.   She told me once that her first husband died in a Japanese POW camp and this explained in some way the kindness of the then Superintendent, when an extra fiver would be included in the expenses of her relatives when they visited her. That would not happen today. The infirm ones sit huddled on a bench seat with blankets round them. Jeannette is in a wheel chair. This time someone has remembered blankets; things must be improving.

I remember the first time I walked round this garden, a couple of weeks after I arrived in 1976, the year of the long hot summer when the girls in Holloway broke all the windows in their old building to let in fresh air. The women in prison, allowed out in the daytime sun, had looked a lot healthier with brown tans, than the pallid psychiatrically cared for women of Broadmoor, allowed fresh air in the weekdays in the evenings only, after tea, when the sun was weaker, lunch-times were taken with staff handovers when there was no movement of patients.   In those days "airing court" was called regularly and everybody had to go into the garden for sometimes several hours, a few walked round, and many complained at weekends at being made to go outside when they were on largactil which reacts to sunlight and causes severe distress; there was little shade, the buildings and three-tiered terraced garden face south to take advantage of the views and sunshine and the shade from the elm trees reflected backwards, onto the house. I walked round with Nan who had been in Broadmoor a few months without striking up a conversation with anybody.

I was her first venture into regaining her memory. She had tried to commit suicide but it was her mother who died of an asthmatic attack trying to save her daughter in the course of which fat from a frying pan had been spilt and Nan taken to hospital to be treated for burns. There she threw herself out of a top floor window fracturing both legs and skull. Her trial had been held without her knowledge; she had been committed as "Unfit to plead". When brought to Broadmoor she had not understood where she was and a nurse had told her: "You murdered your mother didn't you". That alone had been a trauma. "I loved my mother", she said to me, "I couldn't have murdered her". Whenever "airing court" was called and we were counted out most women would sit and chat on the grass or benches but she and I would stroll round together on the path on the middle terrace. She was having group therapy with Dr Murray Cox who had told her that 70% of the women in Broadmoor were in for murder. Whether he had told her this to console her and make her feel more at home with her companions or not was uncertain but the figure certainly preyed on her mind and on that basis at least five in the eight-bed dormitory I was occupying were murderesses. The

pic became so macabre – Nan being almost
bsessed with it she could not believe she was
considered to be what was up to a few years
previously hangable material – that we sat down and
drew up a list to confirm the figures. We did not know
what everybody was in for and made allowances for
ignorance and marked them "M" for murder. One
woman, Nan maintained, had cut off her husband's
willy after having four children in three and a half years
"Murder" we ticked; another had been here ten years,
"She murdered her four children. Her children were by
her father". "I wonder what became of daddy." I
wondered, too, how Nan had acquired so much
information in her semi-mute state. I wonder what
became of Nan. She left years ago after being told by
a social worker from Holloway who came to visit her:
"You're not here for murdering your mother, you know,
but for your suicide attempt". We both wondered if her
records had showed this change of view. She
communicated with nobody here after she left.

I met the ward psychiatrist for the first time a fortnight
after being admitted, Dr Boyce Lecouteur, an
Australian, was on holiday when I arrived. After the
ones I had seen in Holloway Prison I was adamant
that I wanted no more psychiatrists and I had to be
pushed into the office and forcibly sat down in a chair
to meet this one. My first impression was of a hound,
big brown eyes and sunken cheeks resembling a
Basset and Spaniel crossbreed, a sallow complexion
gave him a dirty countenance. I felt him appraising me
in a masculine, not medical, manner and I
endeavoured not to respond. He was a severe
diabetic, requiring two injections a day, on more than
one occasion he had collapsed in a coma at work. I
was told later by a male nurse that "He's the best of

the bunch" and by a female patient, "My parents had to write to DHS to tell him to stop asking dirty questions". A male patient claimed Lecouteur had worked his passage as ship's doctor on the same vessel as he had served and had complained to the shipping company about the stitching of his hand. They had instantly recognised each other when the patient had been admitted to Broadmoor. "You!" each had cried in horror. Dr Lecouteur was responsible for the entire female wing of one hundred and twenty women and a ward on Kent House of around fifty men. One of the conclusions I had reached in Horton with McNeil was that if one psychiatrist was responsible for just one patient no more would be achieved than if the consultant had large case loads but the size of this one did seem excessive. His interviews with me could not be described as in depth. "I didn't want you to come to Broadmoor", he said. I didn't either. He nominated a trainee doctor with a strong Leeds accent to "go over your childhood ailments"; by the second interview we got as far as what my father did in the First World War and then the young man left Broadmoor to continue his career somewhere else.

Dr Lecouteur then asked if I would allow myself to be interviewed at an international conference of psychiatrists to be held at Broadmoor. I agreed. I had nothing to lose but when the day arrived Dr Lecouteur was away on holiday and it was Dr Cyril Levin, the ward MO, who briefed me on the protocol. "You must not mention the name of the hospital or the name of the doctor; merely say 'the hospital' and 'the doctor'". All that happened was that about fifteen psychiatrists of various nationalities, mainly American, took over the ward's non-smoking day room (and smoked) and I sat and recited my case history, Dr Kyp Loucus, RMO on the male side, was Chair. Dr Loucus was the subject of a disparaging *Cutting Edge* programme in 1992. I could not believe any of them would be pleased to hear that a patient had received unnecessary treatment which had caused voices in the head never previously experienced and necessitated three gynaecological operations to counteract the hormone disorders caused by the drugs; what builder is delighted when he hears his buildings have collapsed, but when I had finished and before any of them had a chance to ask any questions Dr Loucus looked at his watch and said, "If we're to catch tea we must go now" and out they all swept.

"What are you doing in OT?" (Occupational Therapy) Boyce Lecouteur would drawl knocking his pipe on the edge of the desk. He was in fact interested in handiwork, did macramé at home and was later delighted with lace making. At regular intervals he whizzed round the various OT sections, which was his form of staff, control, rallying the troops; I imagine he had a diary note to tour the empire once every three months.

Not long after I arrived, Dr Lecouteur embarked on what I was to learn was one of these tours. I was in the OT (which had previously been a large men's dormitory) where all female new admittances started and, if they were not suitable for the other work areas – kitchen, dining room, sewing room and industrial therapy then the only other female work areas - stayed there for the next fifteen or so years. As Lecouteur reached my desk I did not look up from my crochet but I noted he paused slightly before walking on without comment. When we came to pack up, a pair of scissors identical to the one's I had been using was missing.   I was a new girl to searching and did not appreciate the seriousness of a pair of missing scissors.   Ward staff hurtled in to help the search and Sister Jane reprimanded me for not joining in. She was accompanied by the Knicker Picker, a nurse who doubled her duty of searching for unspecified dangerous forbidden objects in our rooms with checking our underwear to see if it required washing. She was so macabre it was said that she dirtied underpants herself merely to assert herself. She regarded me as prime target for bed making and I would be collected out of the OT each morning she was on duty to find my bedclothes littered across the corridor.   She maintained I did not make my bed properly.   I feared both these members of staff; I could not call them nurses. "Can you search round my desk and clear me", I said calmly, "I was using a similar pair of scissors and I think Dr Lecouteur took the pair that's missing".   I was surprised they did not reprimand me for bad thoughts but complied as daylight dawned across the face of Sister Jane.   The scissors were found ultimately in a waste bin that would have been difficult for a patient to reach. It was my first understanding that situations can be created to instigate rules that cannot be qualified by normal circumstances. The rules that were instigated following this incident necessitated signing for tools both in and out.   The capable, motherly woman in charge, May Wear, had resisted the idea as unnecessary.   She was shortly transferred to the female block OT in Lancs House (the Intensive Care Unit), where security was such that even the pins needed to be counted in and out and she had no lovely view but a blank wall to look out on.   It was she who had told me that she had been unable to obtain a pay rise of 15p a week for me for good behaviour and that mention of my name at the weekly clinical team meeting was difficult. May Wear's place was taken by a kindly, affable man, Bill Cerri, who kept a copy of the *Nursing Times* permanently open on his desk at the Situations Vacant column. That such a nice man, with pleasant wife who worked on the ward, could have such a harridan of a mother-in-law (who told Nan she'd murdered her mother and whose husband worked in the Industrial OT, his issue coat fitted with poachers' pockets to remove over two hundred boxes of Christmas cards being packed for the Spastic Society for him to sell privately in a market and anything else that took his fancy) I do not know.

My first visitor was Bill Warwick, a spiritualist whose aim in life was to achieve a spiritual world and whose hearty abhorrence of psychiatry stemmed from his discharge from the Air Force in 1946 through the route of a psychiatric hospital where his tortuous treatment had included ECT without anaesthetic. We had corresponded since 1975 when I included his statement in the petition I delivered to 10 Downing Street appealing for the Abolition of Forced Psychiatric Treatment. I recognised that he had suffered appallingly and that his family had been horrified at his announcement that he was getting married and stepped in to stop the event with the aid of a psychiatrist. He probably had been on a high with delight and unreasonable and the girl of his dreams unsuitable by family estimations but to have somebody committed and literally tortured for being in love takes some understanding particularly when he had served throughout the war to ensure that England was free from such chains. The then ward Charge Nurse was Vic Atkinson, a West Indian known as Aki Paki and heartily disliked by patients and staff alike. "He's been thrown off the male side and dumped on the female wing" I was reliably informed. "He smells," sniffed a nurse, "haven't you noticed we always have the windows open when he's around?" I was concerned that he made mountains out of trivia and wanted to keep me on the ward to talk to me when the others would be made to go out in the garden. I always pleaded that my head did not tolerate much talking – the effect of the drugging by Epsom Police lasted a very long time – and desire for fresh air.

Vic called me to the office, "Do you know a Mr War Wick". "Er?" I said and Vic beamed happily, he was longing to hear that I did not know this gatecrasher. Then I understood, "Warwick", I said, "you pronounce it Warwick" which did not go down well. Mr Atkinson was never wrong and knew everything. He insisted on joining Bill and I on our visit and it took extreme rudeness on my part to get rid of him, he looked set to stay for the full two hours. "Write to Dr Lecouteur and ask him if you can visit Janet", he smiled as he finally got up to leave and I realised this did not bode too well. Bill's stuttering but cheerful gentlemanly demeanour had not influenced the Charge Nurse (I had difficulty in refraining from calling them Charge Hands) on my behalf. The first I knew of the ban was when I was called in to see Lecouteur who had Bill's letter written on lined paper in front of him, "You don't want to know people like this" he said and refused to say why or discuss how my banned visitor was more undesirable than those with whom I came in contact in Broadmoor. Deeply hurt Bill went to MIND who announced they would play the matter "low key". They gave him a letter authorising him to visit me. Broadmoor, once a decision is made stuck to its guns. Bill arrived but was not allowed in. On his behalf

MIND went to the Ombudsman. The result was newspaper items reading: "The Ombudsman upholds banning of unsuitable visitor to dangerous patient at Broadmoor". MIND said they would go to Strasbourg but never did. I had been convinced that Bill would tire of visiting from Stoke-on-Trent and fade away but Broadmoor's ban dedicated him to me and we corresponded till he died. When a patient called Warwick was admitted on the female wing it was conjectured whether her selection for Broadmoor stemmed from her sir name or her crime but neither I nor anybody else took advantage of this to smuggle Bill back in. Another visitor, Niki-Fran who asked me to write her a play, says the visitors' book in Reception states my banned visitor is called Atkins.

Another brave visitor was my sixty-eight year old Aunty Joyce, my Mother's youngest sister, recently recovered from a breast removal through cancer. She arrived looking white and shaken – her arrival at Reception had coincided with a visiting football team of police and a visitor for Ronnie Kray who, although having little to do with him, I always found gentlemanly and courteous. Joyce told me that she was getting married for the first time to a man she had met all those years ago working in Aldenham Castle when she stayed with us during the war.

My first five years in Broadmoor were ghastly because of overcrowding and staff disruption but the years passed quickly because of the fast pace of horror. I was sent to the block (Lancs) twice for no other reason than to create a space for new arrivals and Sister Jane and the Knicker Picker disliked me intensely for no specified reason. They didn't want me on the ward, I was told, and I wondered at a prison that could pick and choose its residents but the experience of being held so low down gave me greater insight to the mechanism of Broadmoor than I would otherwise have received. I was horrified at what I saw and questioned the sanity level of those in authority. My Home Counties English accent was a source for mimic, "Jan. Say fuck off" one young patient had drawled delightedly when we first met and I wondered if the Knicker Picker's Welsh and Sister Jane's half Welsh half Irish background was a problem. I had not been racist before going to Broadmoor; but I now heartily disliked the Welsh and Irish (except for Bill Cerri, his wife etc). After patients on Lancs were left for days without food or water, some with no clothing or pot, there was a radical change in the type of patient admitted.

After five years of chaos, within a fortnight three women arrived with high IQ's, Judith, Joyce and Alvada, with whom I became friendly, and there was a slight lessening in raucous staff behaviour. Although Rampton and Moss Side (later to become Park Lane) specialised in taking those with lower IQ's many of the patients at Broadmoor could be described as difficult because of lack of intellect. Maybe it can be said that those with higher IQ's are less likely to commit mad crimes but this is debateable. Later there was another change with the admission of a succession of very large, fourteen stone was the lightest, coloured women. Staff were clearly frightened of them and it became apparent that these latest inmates received higher doses of medication than the equivalent smaller white patients. The situation did not make for a pleasant atmosphere. Staff paranoia was so intense that on one occasion two of them brought in riding crops, which they brandished at us. What had triggered their fears and actions nobody knew but in all prisons imposing a harsh regime there is an underlying tension.

The Police Force has rules limiting entrants to those of over a certain height; Broadmoor had similar strictures but the shortage of staff and advance of nepotism had allowed this rule to be ignored. There were thus several qualified psychiatric nurses who were barely 5'0" but Napoleon was short and it could be said that the shorter the female nurse the greater the bullshit that emerged. Sister Jane was particularly triumphant one day as she alone escorted a sixteen stone-coloured patient indoors from the garden. We were presently in process of a radical change of patient, one the staff did not like.

The year Lecouteur left through ill health the female wing had a movement rate of six out of a hundred and twenty. That meant an average stay of twenty years per inmate; a visitors' handout stated the general stay to be around four years. In Dr Chandra Ghosh's first year she moved twenty two women thereby proving that the patient's fitness to leave is as much a criteria of the Mental Health Act as the ability and fitness of the psychiatrist and staff to organise that release. Dr Harold Heinson, husband of Dr Chandra Ghosh, was now a psychiatrist at Holloway Prison and he referred patients to his wife at Broadmoor. "Those young thugs you've got on your ward", muttered Joan who had been in Broadmoor thirty five years and witnessed many changes including socials where men sat one side of the room and women the other and allowed to dance but once only with the choice of the opposite sex but this type of admittance was new to her. "They're bad, not mad," she muttered on. I agreed with her. With stories from the male side in mind I added, "Since when has rape been mental illness".

Broadmoor, despite its gruesome reputation, was considered to be a soft option to prison. It had become a place where rules changed constantly and those in need of care and protection were cowed and whimpered.   The new admittances were volatile and retaliated to illogical demands by any means available, mainly verbally, and the staff were clearly nonplussed and angered by what they saw as a challenge to their authority. A large proportion of women were being admitted through the prison, as against the DHS hospital system, and could be labelled psychopaths, a term that sounds horrific when attached to serial rapists but most managements required a large degree of this tendency to manage such an environment. In 1977 female patients could largely be described as docile schizophrenics resigned to being in tears; by 1991 the intake was "young hooligans" determined to get a better deal.   This did not make for good staff relationships and boded far more ill than I could have foretold.

The dim sodium lights from the adjacent land cast shadows through the trees; it was only press publicity on the Governor of Parkhurst who had refused to allow the planting of more lamp-posts in the name of security that had highlighted Broadmoor's greater acquiescence – it had allowed over a hundred more to be situated round the grounds, uprooting flowering almond and cherry trees to make room. A dozen or so had gone into a vacant slope at the back of what had become the Social & Recreation Dept, an area nobody used except the grounds men cutting the grass there twice a year in daylight. It used to be the garden of the

Medical Superintendent and still had remnants of cultivation, a rhododendron flourished amongst the pine trees, a few bulbs pushed their way up in the spring. It didn't take much working out to realise that, if all the over a hundred UK penal establishments each acquired a further hundred lampposts; there would be a rise in the shares of British Steel. Thus I watched my Maggie Thatcher privatisation investment rise after it had sunk by half and I ultimately sold at a small profit, which I would not have had if the Home Office had not intervened. The same exercise with galvanised steel fencing a decade later did not have the same effect and Corus, as Br. Steel became, suffered near liquidation with a £250M loss. The loss would have been nearly £400M without the contribution from Special Hospitals.

"Don't go beyond the summer house" a nurse shouts worriedly that we might somehow disappear into the night. "Oh God", says somebody, "they're treating us like children" and I was reminded of the air raid wardens in my school days during the war; then there was total black-out, no street lighting but we didn't panic like this. War is a good training ground for surviving places like Broadmoor. I was eight years old in 1939 when the Second World War started.

CHAPTER 2 – MY FAMILY BETWEEN THE WARS

My parents married in 1928, their wedding memorable for the vicar who had booked a funeral for the same time and told my parents, "The living must make way for the dead". They had been engaged seven years so another half hour made little difference but that was not the point. They started their married life in Bushey, Herts., which has no particular, claim to fame but symbolised the soul of Britain in the Home Counties and of those times. It was once a feudal village, the remains of a castle were now the British Legion's HQ, and Lord Bethal's estate the offices of a leading insurance company. As a reminder of the effects of war Bushey houses the Royal Masonic Schools for Boys for the sons of deceased masons; the Royal Caledonian School for the children of deceased Scots; St Margaret's School for Girls for the daughters of deceased clergy.   Later the lady bountiful, Mrs Nimmo, would bequeath her beautiful home, Sparrows Hearn on the Heath, to the County for the children of those unable to cope with them.

Pre-war photographs show my mother, nee Myra Tavernor, a teacher, with a group of neighbours, all wearing their husband's cut-down white flannels and waving cigarettes. Bushey might not be on the social map but the inhabitants were making their mark as avante garde. Their generation were heavy smokers and in years to come there was a corresponding cancer toll amongst them. My father, Ernest Coleman, was a government chemist employed at the Building Research Station at Garston. It was his work there that had persuaded him that my mother's dream to move to a bigger and better house was impractical. "There's going to be war with Germany" he announced around 1936, "what I'm working on is military". This was an interesting pronouncement as the country professed to be unprepared to fight three years later.

Most of the relations lived in the Midlands my parents were the rarities of their immediate families on either side to have moved "down South". Visiting relations thus involved a journey and usually a stay of several days, no hopping around the corner to drop in on aunts and uncles for me. When they came to stay with us, the adult relations would expect a tour of London and Windsor, the landmarks becoming familiar to me at an early age; my cousins would visit the Natural History and Science Museums where, in those days, women cleaners would hover round the glass showcases rubbing away sticky finger marks.

Also away from his roots was Uncle Harold, not my father's youngest brother but my mother's cousin. There was a shortage of variety of names in my relatively small family, I had two Aunt Winnie's, two Uncle Harry's, there were two Harold's and forever I was confused with the Liz's. One day, when I was about seven, I was taken to visit Cousin Harold by train, a lovely treat from sitting in the back of a car. You could walk about on trains and there was a restaurant car. On the way there my mother snapped, "Don't go telling him you've been ill. I don't want him practising on you". I had no idea what she meant but I had had whooping cough which had lasted a year and involved a fair amount of lost schooling, nightly chest dressings of smelly Vick, lots of cough linctus, trips to road works to breathe in tar fumes and an operation to remove my tonsils. Today the ailment would probably be diagnosed as asthma. I did not understand that

Cousin Harold Bott was a Christian Science practitioner, turning to the faith following his brother's death from sleeping sickness after returning from India after the First World War; his mother, on her deathbed, had implored Harold to take Christian Science seriously. He did. He threw up his job as headmaster of a boys' school. His father disinherited him but Harold clung to his convictions, visited prisons, built up a clientele and now had a flourishing practice of wealthy ladies on the south coast. He was tall, well built, charismatic and the subject of much gossip amongst the family. He became vegetarian to such an extent that he wore canvas shoes, woollen gloves, used cardboard suitcases and preserved the lives of those wasps that dropped into his stewed apple and custard by fishing them out and setting them out to dry in the sun. With his ability to hold a congregation in thrall and my mother's adeptness to discipline a classroom of over forty seven-year olds in the worst area of Stoke-on-Trent, this was a meeting of Titans.

My mother adored poetry; she came from an era that produced Rupert Brooke's, "There is a corner of a foreign land that is forever England" and fervent patriotism amidst the ravages of war. That era also produced traitors like McClean and Burgess, and fervent communism but Cousin Harold was not political; he had published a book of poems. One of them was dedicated to my mother, the first line reading, "Myra, Myra, how I admire her". Cousin Harold gave us tea in his beach hut on Bournemouth beach. For reasons professional he later changed his name to Harold Carlyon.

Then we had the Mellor's at Enfield, austere, rich, Great-aunt Hagar being my paternal grandfather's sister. She lived till the age of ninety-eight and was old when I knew her. They had one son Ray who ran the family chemist shops. On one occasion my father had called on them to fix their car but his clothing in overalls fit for the job had raised eyebrows and on that occasion he had not been allowed past the servants' quarters. We always wore our best clothes when visiting the Mellors. My mother recounts the only time she laughed at Aunty Hagar's. The old lady had always disliked intensely her brother-in-law, her widowed sister's second husband. Aunt Hagar always referred to him as "That Charles Hill". "What do you think?" she demanded, clutching her black Malacca cane with its silver top. My mother waited patiently; clearly the old lady did not expect a reply. "That Charles Hill has died. And what do you think they have done? They have put him in the same grave. They have buried him on top of her. There is my dear sister Liz lying between the two of them." As Aunt Hagar glared indignantly into space my mother did her best to stop laughing. She nearly wet herself.

I found the Mellor's fascinating for the reason they had a Dalmatian dog called Penny Bun who had a long run in the garden. Penny Bun's mother was stuffed in the Natural History Museum. Strict Baptists, the Mellor's came to view my parents, newly weds at the time, for tea one Sunday. In their own home, not even their servants cooked a meal on the Sabbath. Where most families enjoyed a Sunday roast with cold on Monday, the Mellor's advanced the routine a day.

"You don't have very nice neighbours", old man Mellor's, renowned for sharp dealing in antiques, said. "That man next door is mowing his lawn and it is Sunday, a day of rest."

The neighbours on the new bungalow estate – with long gardens, unmade road, and nearest pub and church a mile away – were perhaps unique in togetherness and community spirit. The husbands had all been in the first war with its toll of a million men so the women were grateful to have a husband at all. The thirties were years of unemployment and depression but everyone in our road had mortgages to pay and all the men had jobs but families were small; some couples were childless. Although not religious, my parents obeyed the traditions and had me christened, presumably to satisfy the relations, particularly the Coleman's.

The man next door, Alf, ex Royal Flying Corp like my father, was my godfather and the woman opposite, Gladys, whose husband Leo had been with the 'Pork and Beans' – Portuguese – one godmother, my father's sister Winnie, the only one who attended church on a regular basis, the other. Alf from next-door and Glad from opposite would walk their dogs at night and it was open knowledge that they were enjoying an affair. Not quite Peyton Place but Little Bushey had its highlights. It was Alf who came rushing back from the village in 1934 with the news that a film was being shot outside Bushey church and I could be in it. I was dressed in my pink organza dress and bonnet, a present from my mother's 'birthday sister' Eugenie, known as Ena (she was born on the same day six years later as my mother), and taken to the village a mile away. I have no memory of my moment of fame but I was told for years afterward that I threw confetti, the name of the film long forgotten but I was in it for a split second and the neighbours went to see it, some went several times as they missed me in the first showing.

When my father built me a doll's house the neighbours combined to contribute items of furniture for it; Aunty Glad made clothes for the tiny dolls inside, her son Dick, then aged twelve, made a chair and so on.   My father made Dick and his friend Geoff pairs of stilts, they all made model yachts and we went in a fleet of cars to sail them on the ponds in front of St Albans Abbey. Dick's had a cabin that filled with water and sunk and he ultimately had to wade into the water to retrieve it. Pops as I called my father, had stitched the two pairs of sails for my yacht himself and for years afterwards oil dripped out when my mother used the Singer sewing machine. I was never allowed to sail the yacht which stood taller than me, it was Pops' own toy made for me, it was stated to be mine and there's a photograph of me with the mast taller than I was, but I was never permitted to touch it.   I was allowed to play with the home made Noah's Ark with its two sets of animals hand-carved in wood, the toy theatre with its two sets of hand-painted scenery and red velvet curtains and of course the dolls' house.   When I outgrew it, the house was given to Jill Davison across the road whose brothers Geoff and Mike converted it into a rabbit hutch. I always envied the Davisons, their sofa sagged and when you pushed it ever so slightly toys cascaded from the back over the floor. Their bread, bought from the same baker, tasted betted than ours. Edna Davison was a bundle of nerves; after Geoff and Mike spent the afternoon cycling on a plank arranged over a cup, the game deemed over when the tea service was devoid of drinking vessels, she picked up her husband's Home Guard boots and threw them. Geoff ducked and there was a broken window to add to the misery.   Geoff later joined the Fleet Air Arm and trained as a pilot but as a teenager the ceiling of the boys' room would be covered with model planes several of which were flown in the field at the back of our garden.   When they lodged in a tree, Aunty Myra's clothes prop would be required to dislodge the toy. The boys would climb into the bottom of our garden and help themselves.   My father made lots of clothes props and my mother drew the line at the removal when it was actually being used to prop up the clothesline.

Pops loved making things.   He was happiest alone in the, later realised to be dangerous, asbestos garage, tinkering with gadgets.   He hand made a cog to make the date function on a grandfather clock inherited when my grandparents died; it didn't work so he made another one that did.   The neighbours were delighted with the crystal sets he constructed in 1928 – the forerunner of radio. Everything worked in our home, although sometimes with a touch of Heath Robinson, probably inherited from the Coleman ancestor who had cut the base off the 1687 grandfather clock when it didn't fit into his low-ceilinged cottage, thereby reducing the value of this valuable heirloom to a few hundred pounds instead of thousands.   I had to grow up and visit other people's homes to realise how useful my father was in practical terms. My first words were reputed to be, "Daddy mend it" and he did remarkable wonders with broken dolls and even soldered wine stems on the work's laboratory Bunsen burner.

We visited my father's family at Christmas. My mother's one attempt at cooking Christmas lunch might have prompted the start of this tradition.   She had purchased a pressure cooker and, typically, had not practised with it beforehand, she saved it till Christmas Day and lunch was a failure of the first order. Uneatable. The purchase had been made on the instalment plan; my parent's only incursion into the never-never and my mother was sued for non-payment.   It was the only occasion she ever appeared in court and when confronted with a demonstration showing that the gadget worked admirably if used correctly she shouted: "It can't be the same pressure cooker. It's a different one". She won. From thereafter we went to the Coleman's for Christmas and crammed into their small house opposite the barracks. This entailed a car journey in the Austin 7 with its leaking soft top to join the annual Coleman family reunion. On Boxing Day 1937 my grandparents took us all to the Prince of Wales Theatre in Birmingham. From a block in the front two rows, where we could see all the make-up, I watched my first pantomime, *Cinderella*. Buttons was played by a young man who was just making a name for himself. George Formby. To this day I can remember him skipping about the stage singing to his ukulele and how sore my hands were from clapping so much.

My grandfather, Philip Coleman, had been a farmer but my grandmother didn't like country life. The story was that she had sat in a cowpat on a picnic wearing a white linen suit and that finished life in the country. There was also a story that she, and therefore all of us, was descended from Francis Drake through her side of the family, the Wheaton line.   The family then moved from Northampton to the Isle of Wight where, at the age of four, my father to the day he died maintained he saw Queen Victoria's funeral procession between two lines of ships stretching from the island to the mainland. "He's inventing it", would hiss my mother, "he can't remember it". Philip Coleman was so Liberal he christened his second son Ewart after Gladstone. Ewart Valentine was always known as Jack and married strict Baptist Winnie who played the organ in church, took the choir, gave private piano lessons and lived till ninety-three. Grandpa also visited parish workhouses in a voluntary capacity and was interested in good works generally. He was never a man to work for others and had a variety of businesses - his firework factory exploded - but when I knew him, he was retired and I had no idea what he had done for a living.

My father always loved fireworks and we would host the neighbourhood Guy Fawkes party, the Catherine wheels fastened to the rose trellis, rockets dangerously placed in upturned buckets – such fun when the buckets flew off with a crash - and the bonfire in the vegetable patch at the end of the garden. Sausages were cooked indoors – it was safer that way. Small children were issued with sparklers, older ones helped plant the rockets and generally assisted to create mayhem with jumping jacks. Today such parties would be banned but there was never an accident at any of ours.

My Aunty Winnie lived with my grandparents and was perhaps typical of her age when one woman in four had no hope of marrying due to the decimation of men in the First War. She worked for the Inland Revenue and would regale with stories of Catholic priests filling in tax returns and inventing families for the Irish working over here. She was strict C of E, the Church, her nieces - four of us - and her parents were her life. She talked and my mother was most unkind about her when detailing either my father or I to take turns to listen to her when she came to stay. Granny Coleman was hunched, adored cards and would frequently survey the prizes at a local whist drive and go and win what she wanted. Her worst win in my lifetime was a booby prize – a very eatable pork pie. If I hadn't been shown photographs of my grandmother as an attractive upright young woman, I would never have guessed that her bent back was caused by osteoporosis. She died of crumbling bones. Of all the relations I resemble her the most and of all the old sepia family photographs the two that stick most in my memory is one (c 1897) of my father aged fifteen months wearing a frilly dress and one taken of the family in 1915. There sit my grandparents with their four offspring, the three boys in army uniform, the expression on Grandma's face speaks worlds. "Come on" she seems to say, "it may be the last time we're together. Smile for posterity". Harold who was younger than my mother, born in May 1900, must have been well under age when he joined up to be with his two older brothers; he became an ambulance driver, surely an experience to make a young teenager mature in advance of his home-based equals. He married beautiful Elsie, five years older than he and they had my cousin Jill.

Each member of the Coleman family played a musical instrument – my father was the flautist – and they held soirees and played chamber music. Forever my father would take the score to a concert and follow every note. My mother did not accompany him. She had different interests. I recall a queue to see the school doctor and my mother enquiring of another mother who was a total stranger to her, "Do you play bridge?" If somebody couldn't play she would teach them. The neighbours were more suited to Newmarket, penny nap and so on which we always played at Christmas, one family playing host to several families, at least twenty people, and play card games for pennies and halfpennies, the scene repeated at another home the next day. Christmas was an exhausting time of year and lasted well into the New Year. But bridge was *the* game.

The Tavernors, my mother's family were quite different to the Coleman's. They were noisier. My mother sometimes took me on the train to stay with them and I always knew we had arrived by the smell of sulphur from the pottery kilns as we drew into Stoke Station. Twenty stone Uncle Nom, Aunty Ena's husband, would collect us in his van that dipped dangerously to one side with his enormous weight. He and Aunty Ena had changed addresses seven times in six years; Aunt E had to decorate and arrange the sale of each house, the accruing profit on each used to buy a shop, which started with pianos. Television was suspended during the war as it interfered with radar but its reintroduction when hostilities ceased made pianos largely redundant as a feature in every home and Couzens became the largest electrical shop in Stoke-on-Trent. At one time Aunty Ena also ran a small shop on a housing estate, Kelvin Stores; Uncle Nom would meet us at the station, drive us home at breakneck speed, cook us all lunch and go back to work where he would entertain other shopkeepers at the back of his shop with the lunch he had cooked there. By the time he left Aunty Ena had still not made the beds, my cousin John was used to it. It was only when widowed did she materialise as efficient in her own right. Uncle Nom was huge and overpowering but he could get anything, despite rationing. Although the

Potteries are industrial and the towns satanic, there is beautiful surrounding countryside with many farms. On one visit my mother went to the bathroom and screamed; a whole salted pig was in the bath – the char lady was not allowed upstairs for six weeks until it was disposed of. From Aunty Ena's we would visit the other relatives mostly having tea in back parlours of small shops as far away as West Kirby. "Napoleon had my family in mind", said my mother, "when he described this country as a nation of shopkeepers". How would he describe it now?

One notable exception to this tendency for self-employment in the Tavernor family was Uncle Harry married to my mother's older sister, Flo. Uncle Harry was manager of the municipal sewerage works; his father had been the Town Clerk, the amount of money he left a cause of a lot of gossip and a count back in the 1920's had showed that thirty-two of his relations worked for the Council. None of the family liked Harry very much; he was a wealth of stories about what people dropped down the drains and wanted back – mostly false teeth   My three cousins, Reg, Joan and Marie were all much older than me so I had little to do with them but Reg was the only member of either side of the family to be on active service during the war; he was an army cook and managed to get back to this country six weeks after the fall of Dunkirk.

The Tavernors, unlike the Liberal Coleman's, were Conservatives to the extent that grandma was Chairwoman of her local party and would appear on stage at political meetings sporting an ear trumpet which I never remember her using at home although my mother maintained grandma was deaf.   Her brother was Governor of the Punjab and it seemed odd that he should have a brother-in-law like Tom, my grandfather who worked in the mines, in those days a dirty business with no pithead showers. In the Potteries it was usual for the bus seats to be filthy and to have a miner returning home from work sit next to you. No wonder my grandmother had a washerwoman who came in daily. In fact grandpa was not a coalface worker but an engineer, and mining engineers get dirty too. His hobby was growing carnations, which nobody was allowed to pick. For some years there was an Alsatian dog that had to be restrained more than previously when my grandmother moved the sofa to find a pile of meat joints. In those days butchers' shops were open fronted which Major found so convenient to augment his dinner.

Then there was Uncle Harry, the only boy of the family with three sisters brighter than him. When my mother started as a student teacher Harry's teacher would come into my mother's classroom to wave her brother's latest show of academic ineptitude in her face. My mother might have gained a reputation for being able to teach other people's children but with her young brother she was not successful and she harboured feelings of insecurity that she should be held accountable for him. Ultimately the other Uncle Harry got him a job at the sewerage works and, after my grandmother died, and my mother persuaded Aunty Joyce (the youngest sister) to leave home, at the age of forty-two he married Nellie, his childhood sweetheart. Aunty Nellie hated me. She did her best to look the same height or shorter than her six foot husband and stooped. "I've come to see my tall aunt", I said after their surprise wedding. She removed all photographs of me from the house. Her conversation and letters were always full of her latest ailments and my mother and Aunty Joyce would conjecture what Nellie would suffer from next.

Most of the children in the road attended Merry Hill School, which required a walk across the recreation ground, a field, and main road. I did not go to Merry Hill; my mother decided I was too delicate to walk in the cold and should travel on the infrequent bus to Oxhey School where she had taught briefly as a supply teacher and admired the headmistress, an austere lady called Miss Oven. Photographs show me as a sturdy child standing on stilts my father made and putting on the back lawn. My father must have loved me very much to have made holes in his lawn for me to knock golf balls into.

When first married my father had not been interested in gardening; showing my mother the property he had opened the back door with the remark, "That's the land" and shut it quickly. Sight of busy neighbours digging away at the field that was their garden – no hiring of rotary diggers then – changed things. As a chemist he applied his knowledge to gardening. There were no garden centres in those days; weed killer and fertiliser, other than manure from the cart horses used by tradesmen, were not mass marketed. My father made up his own prescription to improve his very precious lawn. "What are you doing Mr Coleman?" said Aspidistra Face next door, Grace Brewer, and my father kindly wrote out the prescription for her to take to the chemists. Within days neither had any back lawn at all. So much for home made weed killer of 1936. We would strain our ears to catch what Mrs Brewer would say as she showed her visitors round her garden. We could hear her say, "This came from Hampton Court. This peony I took as a cutting from

Kew Garden and this is from a grave in Bushey Cemetery". She took a large bag and trowel with her everywhere. I was quite young when I realised there was competition amongst the neighbours from the first to hang out the washing on Mondays, hearing the first cuckoo and eating the first home grown crop of peas. I opened the poppies. "Your poppies are out. Mine aren't quite out yet", said Mrs Brewer obligingly but it was years before I told my mother what I had done. I also achieved wonders with a paintbrush on some dahlias.

So to Oxhey School I went, a bus ride away, the bus service hourly. I was eight when allowed to ride to school on my own, which must have been a blessed relief to my mother not to have to collect me at lunch time and take me back again in the afternoon; lunch hours were then two hours to allow for travelling. Oxhey School was a typical Victorian example of the education system with an asphalt playground and outside lavatories fronting a busy road. I can remember my first day there. My mother took me nervously but I was stolid and unemotional, probably had no idea what was happening or what was expected of me. Several children were crying, one boy was yelling for a banana and I gazed in wonderment at him lying on the floor with his legs waving as he screamed. I had never behaved like that in my life; this was a new experience for me. Miss Hammond was my first year teacher; she was lovely with blond hair like mine. The second year was Miss Racket and she was nice too. I was seven when I received a note from a boy in the class, his name was Keith Jewel and he had white hair. The letter said, "I love you". It did not occur to me that he was a clever boy to be able to write me a letter at all; I just did not understand he loved me. With a school teacher for a mother I could read and write before I went to school but did not appreciate I had a head start and did not have to rely on the school to teach me anything for a couple of years. This was lucky as I did have a considerable amount of time off with the so-called whooping cough, which was cured by the removal of my tonsils after which I hardly had a cold for the next twenty-five years.

My mother found a "big girl" to take me to school. One day a man approached us and fiddled with the front of his trousers. The Big Girl went home and told her mother who came to visit mine. My mother was shocked that I had not told her of the incident but it wasn't the sort of thing one spoke about. Nothing happened with the man that I know of so it mattered not if I told my mother anything but I was too young to reason all that out then let alone explain it all.

My father bought his first car jointly with Fred who lived opposite which cost thirty shillings (£1.50) between them; a breakdown lorry brought it and eventually took it away again. In the meantime the two men stripped it down in the field at the back of the garden, put it together again, and learnt to drive it, no driving tests then. The next car cost £3 but the £5 Fiat Tourer took us to Devonshire several times before breaking down on the return journey on the Watford-By-Pass. In Devonshire we camped. My mother was an unlikely candidate to advocate holidaying in a tent but she liked holidays so holidays we had. I can recall vividly my father digging a trench round the tent to allow the floodwaters to drain. It was not all sunshine in the thirties. When not camping in tents we went to holiday camps. I believe the facilities offered to children were the stated reason but my mother enjoyed the tennis and nightlife. My father tagged along and seemed content.

Both my parents had been adults before learning to swim and they were thus determined that I should learn at an early age. My grandchildren passed their 5,000 meters (200 lengths) at the age of 9 but I was delighted with my twenty-five yards certificate at the age of six which, but for Life Saving, I never surpassed. One afternoon a friend's mother took me to Bushey open-air swimming pool, where I slipped from the top of the slide and landed face down on the concrete surround. When I was taken home my Mother passed out at sight of me with chipped teeth, the bits going through my lower lip and blooded nose. Until I encountered a dentist who loved cosmetic dental work I avoided showing my front teeth in photographs; sadly the cappings wore out and I was back to square one until the advent of dentures.

For years my mother had been agitating to move to a bigger and better property but my father's work in the laboratory had told him that war was expected. In 1938 Uncle Jack and Aunty Winnie, both fervent pacifists who practised what they preached, came to stay to attend a Peace Pledge Union rally at the Albert Hall leaving my cousins Muriel and Cynthia with the grandparents. I was eight, in 1939 when Neville Chamberlain had to concede that his statement "Peace In Our Time" of a year earlier was now outdated and announced that the country was at war with Nazi Germany who had invaded Poland. Bushey was thirteen miles north of Marble Arch, five miles from Watford and, although some people were actually evacuated to our area from London my parents thought it expedient for me to go to a remote relative (my father's cousin's widow, Rose Wilcox and her daughter Brenda, aged nine) in an even more remote area in Devonshire, Monkoakhampton.

I was told only that I was going away from the bombs to stay with Aunty Rose I did not really understand what war meant other than soldiers fought each other and planes dropped things. The journey was the slowest of my memory. The Austin 7 had been turned in twelve months earlier and my father had collected from the factory a new Morris 8. We set off in the morning and arrived next day. The roads were packed and we crawled through villages and towns, the worst traffic jam I have ever known; more than half a century later I can remember the lorries full of soldiers across Salisbury Plain and in every town and village the sight of women with rolls of black material under their arms. "Blackout", my mother muttered irritably when I asked what they were carrying and I was none the wiser with the reply. If war achieves anything it can boost the sale of otherwise slow sellers, I can think of no other use than blacking out windows for this drab product. If any housewife bought it in minimum quantity, a few yards at a time I do not know but the ones I saw were staggering with whole rolls of it. We were still some miles from our destination, and the roads beyond Exeter as blocked as those leading to it when we drew onto the kerbside for the night. The owner of a large car parked on the verge in front came up to us and asked my parents if they would like to listen to the news on his car radio. Everyone listened in silence. There was no mirth.

Monkoakhampton could have been a culture shock with its absence of electricity and running water but as a child I accepted in my stride the deficiencies of rural England where all the inhabitants were expected to attend church on Sunday and counted to see who was missing and checked up on later. Aunty Rose was the village headmistress who alternated with the daughter of the manor to play the organ and do the counting to see who missed out on praying. As a child I was expected to join the choir. I couldn't pitch a note, knew it, and stood obediently opening my mouth noiselessly. The old farmhouse, now the schoolmistress' house, stood at the top of the hill, it had "a secret passage" – a servants' stairway, the door to it opening like a cupboard from the kitchen. In later years I could imagine servants creeping down in the small hours to clean the grate and light fires. There was a maid, Vera, who arrived at 5 a.m. with buckets of drinking water she had been obliged to carry across two fields. In the rambling house were Aunty Rose and her 9-year old daughter Brenda, a boy called Warwick related to the other side of the family – he departed to his boarding school quite quickly – my beautiful Aunty Elsie and cousin Jill, three months younger than me, evacuated from Birmingham and Aunty Rose's female companion.

It had been a hot summer and the roof tanks were empty from the drought, which meant there was no water for bathing. As an eight year old this didn't bother me in the slightest, what most delighted me was the conservatory where Aunt Rose, wearing a large veiled hat, spent her time swatting wasps to protect the luscious black grapes. I had grapes for breakfast lunch and tea. Nobody else liked them much. The church school consisted of one room divided by a curtain; another teacher took the younger ones but at eight I was in the big class, I could read and write better than several of the fourteen year olds. On fine days children would not come to school, they stayed helping on their farms, and I was struck how even the youngest could name the birds and wild flowers. There was a milk delivery to the school and the children took home small churns of it for their family's use. At home on top of the hill the main occupation was hanging on the big green gate overlooking the road and watching Vera conducting her affair with the postman.

My mother, who was fond of writing out all my spelling mistakes in my letters to her at the end of her letters to me, never commented that I put too much postage on the envelope. I knew the postage was 1½d if a letter was sent from Bushey to Watford so my logic told me that Devonshire was much further and required more money. I could never check on the postage my parents put on their envelopes as their letters to me were enclosed with their thanks to Aunty Rose for keeping me out of harm's way. It was when I went to the Post Office to buy some sweets and found there weren't any that I wrote asking if I could go home "where the bombs are". There weren't any, and there weren't any sweets in Bushey either, but my father came and collected me and home I went.

My mother was curled up on the sofa in the lounge grinning like a Cheshire cat. The men had been called up and married women were at long last allowed to teach in schools to take the place of the men. The next battle to be won was equal pay but that victory was a long time off. "My country needs me", said my mother grinning broadly. How she could be happy teaching no less than forty-five seven-year old boys, one year she had fifty, at Merryhill School is a mystery to me. From three weeks before the end of each term she lost her voice completely. The country also needed my father who moved laboratories several times before being settled into a large country house with Adam ceilings and large stables near Leamington Spa. He served in the Home Guard both home and away and appeared alternate weekends, the limit of his petrol allowance, to spend his time in the garden to "Dig for Victory". He grew all our vegetables. On one occasion he was digging away when Leo from opposite called. "Oh come on Ern", he said in his attempts to get my Dad to take part in Home Guard manoeuvres, "we're playing the real army". Not exactly renowned for an encouraging attitude towards the endeavours of others, my mother would say of the Home Guard, "My God. If we're depending on your father and that lot we might as well give in now".

The war and doing her bit teaching gave my mother reason to employ a daily who came twice a week. The first woman was tiny but could move the piano unaided, the one I remember most objected to being left notes what to do, the words, "Rub hard" particularly annoyed and there was a very noisy row but my mother was determined not to lose her even though she needed help to move the piano on which I reached Grade III with my rendering of *Fur Elise*. I developed a dislike of dailies and resolved never to employ one. Why pay somebody to come and do your housework when you had to do it all first to have the house nice and tidy for fear of what the help would gossip about.

For a while I failed to understand that whilst I had been at school in rural England the local schools had been closed. Thus I had been denied a holiday. I felt quite cheated but did not stay much longer at Oxhey before passing the entrance exam to Watford Grammar School for Girls. If I had not passed I was told I would go to Rosary Priory, a Catholic establishment, "Where they teach you to sew". My mother's views on education were firmly established; brains were educated academically, those less endowed with grey matter did needlework. "Girls 6 – 18: Preparatory for Boys" said the notice board outside the Priory which my mother would take visitors to read and laugh at. I was shy and bit my nails.

I cannot imagine what I would have been like with atheist/agnostic parents and having to attend a strict Catholic school.

I had not been long at Watford Grammar School where the juniors were situated in Lady's Close, a house near the main school building, when the air-raid siren went. We were marshalled into the basement cloakroom where a large jar of barley sugars was handed round and we sang songs. It was quite nice. It never happened again. Our teachers were spinster ladies dedicated to our education and the Germans were not going to disrupt our lives like that. From then on a scheme was devised whereby we had three minutes. The air-raid siren was treated as a warning but we took no notice of it unless a hooter sounded and then we ran. On two occasions we weren't all in before the All Clear went but we were not concerned, we developed a blasé attitude towards what the Germans were trying to do.

Such dedication to our education was in contrast to the dictum of the Principle who maintained that we should compete against ourselves and not against each other. To this end we had no exams; my mother was one of several parents who protested to no avail and the policy was reflected in the School Certificate results of some years hence when twenty five percent of the girls failed. The boy's grammar school on the other hand, decimated of male staff and manned with women who hadn't taught for years, the elderly brought back from retirement and crippled young males had only two failures over a five year period which was a remarkable achievement.

The school had five hundred and fifty girls when I started there in 1940; when I left in 1948 there were eleven hundred; that there was not chaos in between shows an iron discipline and skill at organising. Although it was odd having French in the stationery cupboard and evacuating to the dining room when hockey was cancelled in bad weather and other classes occupied our classrooms, there was extraordinary calm throughout the war years. In retrospect I admire those teachers enormously. The main building was situated next to Benskin's Brewery and, when the wind blew from that direction, the smell could be overpowering so the windows had to be closed. I don't recall the classrooms being stuffy. I do remember the cold. The central heating was Spartan during the war years and wearing an overcoat was frowned upon and unheard of. We did wear vests and liberty bodices and thick black stockings that schoolchildren today would scorn.

I can still see my mother sobbing over the radio, our mainstay. She listened to the news and cried at announcements of shipping losses and German advancement across Europe. She cried throughout an Empire Day celebration held in her schoolyard with the children waving Union Jacks and singing, "There'll

Always Be An England". She had told me, but it did not sink in at the time, about the soup kitchens of the First World War and how boys with whom she had been at school joined up on leaving and were dead in six weeks. Despite being an escapist in many ways, my mother had an unusual streak of realism. She was not like Uncle Jack's Winnie who spent the entire war without once listening to the news or reading a newspaper but devoting her time to her two daughters, my cousins Muriel and Cynthia, music at the Church and giving private piano lessons. The trouble was that my mother did not disguise what reality did to her. She cried.

The local ARP (Air Raid Precaution) man was Mr Rutherford. If he saw a chink of light showing through the curtains he would knock at the door and shout, "Turn that light off". I think he enjoyed doing it. He had three daughters and a gun. "If those Germans come I'm going to shoot my girls. I'm not going to let those Jerries rape them", he announced. At least my parents did not put me through the horror of imagining what it would be like to die at the hands of my father protecting me from the unimaginable. Whilst the Battle of Britain raged we fully expected Germans to parachute into the fields at the end of the garden to secure Watford By-pass en route to London.

As pre-war my father had worked at the Building Research Laboratories, where radar was the top-secret discovery and housed in an old shed, he knew the best air-raid shelter to get. Thus several concrete slabs were delivered, cost £22, and a large hole dug in the garden to house them. A man was called in to help dig the hole. Bunks were constructed inside the shelter and my mother and I were thus safe from bombs. My mother was lonely with my father away and when her youngest sister, Joyce came to stay for two weeks as a break from looking after her widowed father and brother who were unused to helping in the house, she persuaded Joyce to stay for the next four years. My Uncle Harry solved the problem of housekeeping by marrying Nellie. My mother taught Joyce to play bridge and the latter got a job with an insurance company which had evacuated from St Paul's to Aldenham Castle, some five fields away. This was a change from being a bookkeeper at Wedgwood, where no washing up was done for the tea breaks – china seconds were used and broken after use.

Although the siren went when war was declared it didn't go again for some time. When the raids did start, mainly in the evening we would troop into the shelter and troop out again when the all clear went. After a while we stayed put and slept, not knowing in the morning if the raid was still on. However, it was not long before the habit was given up completely as the shelter filled with water and became a reservoir to nurture the garden. The man who had dug the hole for the shelter was called back and the precious lawn was dug up to lay drains, which made no difference. In future years I came to believe that this flooding saved my life – I would surely have developed a serious lung condition from the fumes generated by my mother and her sister's smoking without my father's contribution to the fug. My father, home one weekend, assessed the situation and was adamant that the casters be removed from my bed, which was then jacked up on blocks but my mother, refused to allow her divan to be treated similarly. Although she could panic over trivialities like my standing on the table to reach something she was pragmatic about being killed by a bomb. Thus I slept under a bed for two years and would usually awake each day unaware of the night's activities. I slept like the proverbial log except once. It was under my bed that I was awakened one night to a reverberating swoosh and a big bang which shook the building. My father was home at the time. "That was near" he said as he and my mother rolled out of bed. "Oh", said my mother, "it's like that all the time". In the morning we opened the back door to find the garden littered with large clods of earth. The bomb was a land mine; in those days a land mine was a large time-bomb, descending by parachute and designed to explode after the raid was over; this one had had slipped its moorings; the milkman would come round with bits of parachute material for women to make underwear. The bomb landed in the field at the bottom of the garden and the crater it made was large enough for me to learn to skate on when it filled with water and froze over in 1947. I wore some detachable skates that had rusted in the garden shed since 1928 and stuck them onto Pops' Home Guard boots padded out with three pairs of oiled sheepskin socks. I was towed on the end of a scarf by a boy friend, John Perry, who I met cycling to school with his friend David.

One day when the news was particularly grim my smiling father came to my bedroom and said to me under the bed; "It's all right. We're going to win. Churchill's taken over". With my mother hovering in the background whimpering, "He's mad", he continued, "he turned the tide in 1915 and he'll do it this time". He must have been the only person I knew who thought we could win against the German invasion but on this occasion he displayed one of his peculiar flashes of insight which some took for naiveté and false hope. At school the disappearance of those of

German origin when Churchill came to power and reappearance when hostilities ceased was treated without comment. The girls had been detained with their families on the Isle of Man.

I sat next to Barbara who explained her absence from school the previous day with: "I saw a psychiatrist", she was clearly embarrassed and shifted uneasily. I had never heard the word before and tried to look knowledgeable.

"It's about my asthma", she continued, "They think it's because I'm worried about things at home". I still did not understand, I hardly knew what asthma was but I did know that Barbara was one of six, their mother, who was a housewife and had no outside job, looked careworn and I had seen their youthful-looking father taking several of his family to play tennis on the local recreation courts. All the children were clever, the family poor by weight of numbers. My family would have been poor if there had been six instead of one of me. Barbara was worried by the interview with the psychiatrist of German Jewish origin, with whom she had spent the afternoon playing board games. She did not like him at all. She found him creepy. I don't think she attended the clinic again – it involved missing her schooling - and today it is indeed ludicrous that asthma can be regarded as psychosomatic and curable with a chat and Ludo. I did not appreciate that Hitler had disliked psychiatrists on the grounds that many refused to sign extermination papers for the mentally disabled so not only Jewish ones had fled to this country for refuge or that work was being created for them. I did not appreciate that psychiatrists were a law unto themselves and that Hitler was responsible for the UK having more of them per head of population than any other country. Many of them, including Freud, settled in Hampstead, which claimed at one time to have the most psychiatrists and the highest mental illness rate in the UK. There is a moral to this correlation somewhere.

Holidays at grammar schools were longer than Council schools so I would frequently be obliged to accompany my mother to her school. School dinners had become universal; they removed the necessity for mothers to stay home from the factories to cook and lessened the risk of children travelling during raids. I therefore had to take lunch with the teachers in the Parish Hall up the road and afterwards, to utilise my presence I frequently read to the boys from the books my Mother purloined from me in the interest of the war effort while she balanced the dinner money, these days duties performed by the school secretary which post did not then exist. I had a beautifully illustrated copy of *Alice In Wonderland*, which was a favourite with the boys and *The Wizard of Oz*, which was approved by my mother as a lesson in self-determination as the characters overcame their difficulties by their own endeavours. The cowardly lion found he was brave after all, the scarecrow that he did have brains and so on. I don't know what she would make of today's *Lord of the Rings* where the characters rub a ring to escape their difficulties. Too easy. My father made her education aids, cards with pictures, A for Apple, B for Ball. My Mother estimated that a third of the children moving from infant to junior school could not read or write and without reading children could not do arithmetic. She claimed to have taught every child who went through her hands something. At the age of 16, long after he left, one boy would call into the school as he passed and draw an animal on the blackboard, write the word 'pig' and go off again clutching the penny she gave him. It was the only word he learnt at school. There was a serious downside to the nation's need of my mother in the education system; she became so used to controlling over forty boys that I would find her overbearing and I was required to wipe up and do the shopping. I had more pocket money than most in the class but I earned it. My Mother would pay me so much a week and Pops so much a month for mowing the lawns and keeping the hedges clipped.

My mother could not ride a bike. She had no sense of balance – but could play tennis and badminton. Her attempts at learning to drive a car resulted in her screaming when a bus approached on its own side of the road. Thus my ability on a bike, and my father's competence at maintaining it made me, and later Joyce as well, a candidate for the shopping. "It's not far on your bicycle", my mother would say, displaying her unarguable logic, when requiring me to go into the village.

Although the practice of milk delivery at 6 a.m. and another later in the morning had been reduced to one delivery only, milk and bread were delivered right through the war. As we were out, stones had to be put on top of the milk bottles to stop the starlings pecking at them. The milkman was a member of the RSPCC, his job enabling him to check on child abuse but I never heard of him reporting anybody in our area. He kept the Co-op number written in pencil on the frame to the back door so he did not need to check it each time the bill was paid. It was not possible, however, for the butcher to deliver the tiny portions of meat ration. As things were, tradesmen received grants to compensate in some way for the loss of revenue and increased paperwork with food tokens. The butcher – phone number Bushey Heath 1940 – was on top of a steep hill and on Saturday mornings I would walk up it to collect the meat ration for us and two other families of old people who could barely walk, let alone get as far as the butchers and coast downhill again. I never remember either family thanking me for my services of errand girl. My delivery of the week's meat ration would always be greeted with: "Is that all?" A shilling a week, plus a penny's worth of corned beef, would purchase one chop or equal which meant that cheap cuts which went furthest would top the priority list; Sunday lunch would take several hours to cook as the gas pressure was so low. The gas was never turned off as in those days it was dangerous when it came on again but however severe the bombing the gas supply stayed on, however low the pressure. After London docks were bombed, we could see the sky glowing red for a week and food rationing became more severe, the tea ration cut. Although hoarding was frowned upon, our cupboards had been stocked full since prior to the declaration of war. Items like bags of sugar, tea and tins of salmon, fruit and soup were stacked high. Niceties, or impediments, like 'sell by' dates and bar codes had not been invented and so long as the ingredients didn't smell off they were eaten. I never recall any incident of food poisoning.

At school our Headmistress, Eton cropped Jean Davison, announced at assembly one morning, "You must remember that the children of Europe are starving, they have no food at all, and it is regretted that the standard in this school will not be as we would wish. An Oslo Breakfast will be served in the Cookery Room and pupils will partake on a rota every three weeks. This will consist of a jacket potato and salad. And there will be more milk puddings". Ugh. I loathed all of it. My mother would cook my father a rice pudding on Sundays while she and I would have apple pie and custard. Unannounced by Miss Davison were the sausages. Whale meat sausages. They were the worst sausages, the second most revolting being Broadmoor's beef sausages when I first went there, and it says something for my mother that we never had them at home however nutritious they might be. The Oslo thing was an example of the attempt to provide children with healthy food, which the children did not appreciate. As it was I took to sneaking my disliked nutrition onto a ledge beneath the trestle table in the dining room but had a panic and took along my shoe bag to empty the debris into when I heard the room was to be used for a parents' meeting. My mother refused to provide me with sandwiches, she said she had nothing to put in them and frequently I had no food at all day rather than eat the muckarelli, as I called it, provided for school lunch.

Fish was not rationed so there was invariably a queue at the fishmongers. To this day I have a picture of a line of women, some with scarves to cover their curlers, all with drawn faces, my mother's among them. None laughed or made a joke although the bravery of the fishermen to provide the catch was probably forgotten. What was on offer on the fish slabs was sometimes a motley collection of marine life but, even at the height of shortages, my mother was selective. We had turbot and halibut, (now prohibitively priced), plaice and sometimes smoked haddock or kippers. It is amazing that cod is now in short supply, prized and over-fished as my family did its best to preserve it. They never bought it. My mother was like the apprentices in Dickens' day who objected to salmon as too everyday. Cod was taboo.

Rationing bit hard but it says something that we did receive what we were allocated; the nadir was 1 oz butter and one egg a week but in times of "plenty" we would preserve what we could. Eggs went into a metal bucket of isinglass to be used for cooking or omelettes – we never boiled preserved eggs - potatoes were stored in sacks, onions strung up, runner beans salted in a wooden barrel all stored in the garden shed. Forever I can recall the difficulty of rinsing out the salt – bought in large blocks - when the beans were scooped out of the barrel, salt was never added to the cooking water and still they tasted over-seasoned. What fruit we could obtain we bottled in Kilner jars and there was an allocation of sugar for jam making. We even used the tiny fruit on the Siberian crab tree for blackberry and apple jam. Bought jam had a terrible reputation with stories of wood chips for raspberry pips and the bulk made up of turnips so we always made our own. Forever I can remember sitting in front of the fire de-pipping sultanas and raisins for the Christmas cake and the mincemeat. It was an incredibly sticky job and I doubt would pass any health and safety regulations. The wonderment at buying dried fruit with the pips removed was unheard of and I hope the man who invented that one reaped the benefit he deserved.

Coal was limited. It was still readily available in the coal-mining areas but the allowance in Bushey was 1 cwt, a sack, when the coalman came round with his dray-pulled cart. It became habit, therefore, to buy coal all the year round, even in a heatwave, to store for the winter, sometimes we had difficulty storing it, the surplus would overflow the coalbunker onto the patio.

Even then a brick was put in the fireplace so less coal was used. For my mother brought up in a mining area with free coal to pit workers this was sheer purgatory, the brick an offence. Roaring fires were an essential, not that miserly little glimmer in the hearth.

Sometimes my father would take me back to Leamington with him and his landlady would look after me. She was very kind. Her daughter had died so I had to be careful and not spoil the children's books and toys in my room. His idea of entertaining me was for us to go to the Globe Theatre at Stratford where we saw the comedies. He adored the Marx Brothers and Mae West.

The parental habit of becoming emotional when running out of cigarettes had made me interested in what there was about smoking that made it a necessity. The worry of running short had produced the custom of having a box of fifty or hundred Passing Cloud or Players Senior Service, whatever was in vogue and available at the time, in the dining room, bedroom and breakfast room… In addition, both parents carried cigarette cases. It was inevitable that one afternoon, when I was barely nine and my mother was out, a girl friend and I sat and tried our luck. The dog ends we threw out of the window onto the flowerbed bordering the pathway to the front door. There were a lot of dog ends but the wrath that followed was totally unnecessary. I am a confirmed non-smoker for the sole reason I got nothing out of it. With each increase in the duty on cigarettes my mother would declare: "I've smoked since I was fourteen and no Chancellor of the Exchequer will make me give up". She also stated that her cigarette smoking and income tax which was 9s.6d. in the £

(45p today) paid for the war. Such wild assertions were typical of her.

It was lucky my mother liked walking; even if she could drive a car there was strict petrol rationing for official use only but we would go blackberry and mushroom picking not only in the nearby fields but take the bus to Chandlers' Cross, beyond Watford, where she and my Aunty Joyce would have a beer sitting outside the pub and I a lemonade. It was on one of these excursions that a heavy drone distracted us; the sky and the sunny fields went black as the shadows of Dakotas towing gliders flitted over us like an omen of foreboding. The darkness did not last a minute or two, but ages, an hour or more. The sky was covered with planes. The drone went on and on. This was the start of the Battle of Arnham; unbeknown to us one of our neighbours was sitting up there waiting to jump into the arms of a crack division of German Panzers.

In the evenings, when there was no bridge party – my mother had been known to host one in the afternoon and attend another in the evening - I would often be urged to finish my homework and we would go to the cinema; this could happen twice or more a week, depending how bored my mother was, and what was showing. More than once we missed the last bus and would have to walk the five miles home. I would never have believed that over fifty years on these films would be viewed from a box in one's own home. They might appear dated now but I can recall seeing them when they were first issued and how they inspired and uplifted. We cried at *In Which We Serve*, Noel Coward's film of the Royal Navy; *Mrs Minerva* was us, a life to which we could relate. Propaganda these films were then, with the enemy clearly depicted, the

English serviceman always the hero, and we queued gladly to see them. There would be a B movie too and the news, the only opportunity we had to see animated accounts of the war, which affected all of us. We often went to the Watford Rep, Alan and Winnifred Melville were the stars – the life of a repertory actor then was to perform the current week's play, rehearse next week's and read the lines through for the week after.

It sounds terrible now to say it publicly but we cheered when Germany invaded Russia and the Japanese bombed Pearl Harbour. England was no longer alone in her struggle against Germany. After America came in to the war, and prior to D-Day there were a million US troops stationed in the UK. Bushey Hall Hotel became a base for the American army and as I cycled home from school one day I was surprised to see a row of GI's sitting on the wall whistling as I rode past in my school uniform. Their numbers made the cinema queues much longer. Watford also had Dutch and Canadian troops. Nobody knew what they were all doing. Bushey Heath was deemed a security zone with Bentley Priory for the RAF's Bomber Command, Anti-Aircraft Command and so on. We did not appreciate that the area was that important. It was a nuisance for some Belgian friends of ours who lived on the Heath, the wife's sister was deemed an alien and not allowed to visit them; they would meet in Watford four miles away.

At the time of the guided missiles, the Doodlebugs, V1's and II's, the siren would go off frequently; one afternoon my mother and I were at the cinema and we counted how many times a notice reading "The Air Raid Alert Has Sounded" appeared on the screen. It included a homily about the cinema's shelter and air raid personnel taking their posts and it appeared twenty six times. Not a person moved. The notice announcing the all clear also appeared twenty six times and it was all greeted with derision and clapping by the audience. I can't remember what the film was called.

We became very blasé and I would exaggerate events for the benefit of our, particularly my mother's relations who didn't know what a bomb was from personal experience, and other girls at school whose experiences in North Watford were greater than mine and I did not wish to be missed out. The events there were I seemed to miss. I came home from school one misty late October to be met by a policeman standing at the bottom of Chiltern Avenue, parallel to the road where I lived. "Where are you going?" he asked

"Home" I replied and he asked me where that was.

"Oh that's all right", he said, "but don't go near number...." I forgot what he said; I don't think I even heard him. When I arrived home my Mother, still in her overcoat and fur-lined boots, cigarette in mouth, had just finished lighting the fire. The living room window was open. I went to close it. "Oh leave it", she said gloomily, "the police have been round. We've got to leave all the windows open. There's an unexploded bomb in the Gascoigne's garden. They've been evacuated". The Gascoigne's garden fronted the sleeper track I had used to walk home. I had walked right past the bomb and not known it. I didn't feel a sense of relief that it had not gone up as I walked past but a feeling of being cheated of some excitement but I admired still more the bomb-disposal squads whose job it was to make the missiles safe.

Both my parents came from families sceptical of tales of the supernatural, Grandpa Philip was famous for exposing one illusionist with a torch in the middle of a séance but they found it difficult to find a pragmatic explanation for the story Joyce brought home after a visit to a séance in Watford, taken there for fun by a work colleague. "Have we an aunt who lived in the country?", enquired Joyce of my mother.

"Aunt Lizzie" was the reply. "She died before you were born. She lived in the country and had a two holer…."(a privy for two. Even by 1945 a quarter of all houses in the country had no inside lav).

"…because she sent a message to say Flo needn't worry about Marie. It will be all right." Cousin Marie had announced she was marrying Adib, one of the Palestinian soldiers stationed in Stoke. "He'll have four wives and you'll be stuck in a tent", the family had cried but the couple were adamant. Later, after the war, Adib returned to Palestine, settled his affairs, went down the coalmines as a condition of gaining entry back into this country, and married Marie. They were never rich but he was a good husband and Marie his only wife. In later years it seemed very sad that Israel treated the Palestinians so shabbily when they had supplied a regiment to fight to liberate the Jews from Hitler's Germany. How short are memories. How full circle history flows in time.

I was in the village one afternoon and due to join my mother at her school later when a noise in the sky stopped; I looked up to see a doodlebug (VI) quietly poised, its puffing engine had run out of fuel. You could stand and watch doodlebugs puffing across the sky but when the engine stopped was another matter. I was mesmerised and stood staring. A man on the opposite side of the empty street saw me looking and looked up too. "Get down", he roared and I lay flat on the pavement. Out of the corner of one eye I could see the flying bomb dip towards me, level up and lift itself above the shops. It was a second or two before it crashed. The "whoomp" brought out the shop windows for the second time in six weeks and killed a sheep and a crow in the Moat Field. ARP Warden Mr Rutherford met my friend Brian on his way back from collecting a souvenir of smouldering shrapnel from the crater: "Where was it boy", cried Mr Rutherford wobbling on his bike. "The Moat Field", says Brian. "Get under cover boy. Get under cover", the ARP man shouted as cycled on to survey the damage. I picked my way through the broken glass; already appearing in shop entrances were notices stating, "Business as usual". It was good experience for surviving the psychiatric system.

CHAPTER 3 - BROADMOOR

After the All Clear

After the fire engine departed we trouped indoors to the same counting procedure as on the way out.   Liz was put in seclusion. Times have changed. When I first came here in 1976 she would have been sent to the Block immediately without consultation with the doctors, the opportunity welcomed to make one less on the ward, the space to be filled very soon by a new admission or an optimist promoted from the Block.   If staff or patients disliked the newcomer her stay on York II was short-lived and back she would go to Intensive Care, there was no tolerance for those of a nervous disposition.   Over the years I had experienced to my detriment three nurses undergoing nervous breakdowns due to their own personal problems; I never knew one member of staff go under with the stress of the ward but many patients did.

I filled in the rest of the evening playing canasta with Babs, "Sorry I'm so slow", she said. The ward's unsettled. Jo's on the Block. Judith swallowed a battery, the Annual Show's next week, these and other disturbing influences were shut out as the act of playing cards provided an anchor to which my mind could return when required.

"Have you always been like it?" I asked, expecting her to say, "it's the drugs".

"Since my lobotomy. I had aggression cut out. Didn't you know?" No. I hadn't heard. Twenty years ago she attacked everyone who came near.   What a lot of tragedies are caused by accidents of birth. She's determined "they" want us out. I need convincing of that one. I'm trying to take my mind off a case conference a week ago. My friend who came to it had met two representatives from SHSA (Special Hospitals Service Authority) and one from the Home Office tumbling out of a car outside. One of the SHSA men had been chanting like a mantra ticking off his fingers as he sat in the waiting room, "Is she dangerous? Is she a danger to the public? Is she a danger to herself?" He was talking about me. Also there was a probation officer from Hereford who said he had eleven murderers from prison on his books, not one requiring as many interviews and visits to Broadmoor as me who hadn't killed anyone. After seeing the character assassination called medical reports I had developed a cynicism that the conference, the tribunal and so on were merely camouflage to keep me in and conceal still further the questionable peculiarities of the medical profession. If the psychiatrist, Chandra Ghosh, wanted me out, as my Hereford friend who I would live with maintained, and who has formed such a friendship with the shrink that it is jeopardising her friendship with me - she gives the ward psychiatrist a lift on Fridays when she visits and has got very pally - then why aren't the recommendations for discharge more positive. Psychiatrists have ruined my life; I do not want my friends being friends with them.

A group of us were coming back from the dentist situated in the Medical Centre, when we met the Social Worker, John Waters, on the stairs. "When are you going to Hereford?" I enquire. "After I've seen you", he replies in his Wiltshire burr. "When's that?" I ask. "When it's convenient", he says, "when I've been upstairs". Half an hour later he was telling me, "You don't think you're going to get out quickly, d'yer?

78

There are more reports; I have to contact your daughter and Dr Ghosh has to collate all those reports in one file".

"Her Secretary can do that" I said, my heart very low. I have already been here fourteen years. He is depressing but I had long ago learnt that optimism in the psychiatric world leads to disappointment. He had asked no relevant questions to a discharge. No questions how I would establish my identify, no questions if I had a bank account, how I would manage financially, or give some indication how much State benefit I could expect. He had not even enquired if I had anything to ask him. I gauged he was not relishing his trip to inspect my friend's premises – a Grade III Georgian listed property with large grounds. His predecessor had intimated that people who owned such properties had acquired their money dubiously, probably from the slave trade or opium dealings with China, and that I was regarded by my friend as a conscript for her chores. I certainly expected to help my friend, I could not expect her to board me for nothing and do nothing to contribute to the running of her household. I found the inference offensive but this social worker seemed even worse. Did released IRA terrorists have their homes inspected prior to discharge? There would be a revolt if that happened. The interview petered out and I am left wondering what the purpose of it was. Not for the first time I wondered how much benefit patients and their relatives derived from social workers and their reports, which seemed to be compiled to qualify the existence of the reporter. It was rather like donations to Oxfam where most of it is spent on administration and the drought-stricken natives stay thirsty.

Mitch has wandered over to see who's winning at our canasta. "Nobody in the smoking day-room knows if Germany was one country before the war", she says and I understand that she does not know this either and is asking me. Ignorance comes in many guises and is deceptive; I may know that Germany was once one country but I could not recite the members of pop bands or their hits so I am a dimwit to many who are labelled dim by me. "Liz's been taken downstairs. Vera's unhappy", Vera was Liz's friend and Liz of the fire bell pressing to get a headache pill had shown both of us a copy of the letter Liz's husband had written to Broadmoor saying that Vera, Liz's friend, was a bad influence. The fire alarm incident had provided a good reason for Liz's transfer to the ward downstairs which is better than this one on the first floor but the transfer is strange, displays a complete change of policy. Nobody has ever been promoted for being a nuisance. I was on the ward downstairs and content there until the use of the main dining room in an adjoining building was abandoned and eating facilities created for each ward. This prevented the necessity of ward movements at meal times; it also prevented my eating in York I's dining room, as the noise from the fan-freezer and my tinnitus did not make for comfortable dining particularly as we had to wait till everyone was finished eating and the cutlery counted in and found correct. I was demoted and sent upstairs where I had to start from scratch in the dormitory, which was dreadful. I was scared and felt a slight reprieve when a friend brought me in a pile of eats so that I could arrange a dormitory feast, thereby breaking the rules but gaining favour with the tough girls whose moods changed quickly from being pleasant to pulling hair out in handfuls for no apparent reason. I daubed prawns with garlic dressing on

Swedish bread rolls and hoped our breath next day would not give the game away and we could dispose of the crumbs. The difference between Liz being promoted and I demoted was that Liz's move stemmed from her complaining about staff's refusal to give her a pill; my move stemmed from tinnitus caused by the psychiatrist's forcing medication. This was a reason I was sceptical that I would be released; if the psychiatrist had promoted instead of demoted me I would have more faith.

The staff-in-charge were patently sympathetic and, after a few weeks, offered me a job of ward worker, which went with the best room on the ward. It was twice the size of most rooms and had been the night staff's bedroom in the days staff slept over. It had been wallpapered some fifteen years previously in yellows and orange that had faded. Usually rooms were painted and in most the paint had peeled leaving bare patches, in this room chunks of wallpaper were missing. I pushed the wardrobe in front of the largest torn gap, the dressing table was also strategically arranged and I put some photographs and a calendar over the other worst patches. Whereas graffiti had been a feature of prison cells at Holloway here it was not allowed and some semblance of decency pervaded. Not much. But some. At Holloway cockroaches had been taken for granted; at Broadmoor they were reported and dealt with. It was a mixed blessing when the entire house was refurbished, including the roof. We would be transferred to a vacant ward on the top floor, the occupants of that ward being transferred and refused to come back again. They stayed on the ground floor of a men's block for thirteen years until they were ordered back to York House.

81

Our staff had decided they could not take our increased freedom from the new management any more and set about to reduce the amount of our belongings by the means available to them. These included exchanging our wardrobes for smaller ones and imposing rules whereby we could stand nothing on top of them. The Estates department who supplied the furniture were clearly cognisant of the arrangement. Some terrible scenes ensued. Some of the more vocal women were given parole to shut them up. I still did not have parole. Parole in prison is different to Broadmoor where it means little more than the acquisition of a cigarette lighter during the daytime and the ability to go unescorted to the shop, or canteen as it is called, at stated times when the usually locked gates would be unlocked. I do not smoke and I am not a heavy shopper at the canteen. Not for me a dozen large bottles of Coca Cola, "I have to drink a lot. It's the drugs make my mouth dry" or packets of crisps and Pot Noodles. At one time Broadmoor was the largest outlet for Old Holborn tobacco.

When the men's houses were refurbished they were allowed to take as much as they wanted with them to their new or temporary abode whereas female staff literally fought to make our possessions go into three paper sacks. I cheated and slipped up the stairs carrying another one. It was a temporary respite. If the tactics used had not been so underhand and a more open statement made of staff difficulties a great deal of distress would have been avoided. As it was, the tension increased and some female staff refused to work on the ward thereby earning it a bad name. The situation continued for several years, and manifested itself in an enormous amount of verbal abuse and window and crockery smashing to the extent that the glass windows needed to be replaced with plastic at considerable expense and the number of those "cutting up" increased dramatically. There had been very little of this when I first went to Broadmoor in 1977, by the time I left in 2003 so many women had serious cut marks across their arms and legs it could be regarded as tribal practice.

The room furnishings today are smarter in appearance now than they were twenty years ago but house far less; the beds are fixed to the floor with steel bars making it nearly impossible to clean beneath, the wardrobes are built-in and fixed as are the dressing tables – all are open-fronted, none have doors so the possibility of suicide by hanging is reduced. Comfort and hygiene out of the door. Hardly anybody has a chair to sit on and, with some staff on some wards, lying on the bed is forbidden except at appropriate times. Women write letters and do their homework for the Education Centre kneeling on the floor in their rooms. It is impossible to have a four at canasta these days – there is a dearth of tables and moveable chairs. At one time, on the Block which imposed greater security, there would be several games of canasta going, staff joining in shift after shift which helped staff/patient relationships provided losing was not taken too seriously. There were never any instances of chair throwing. The absence of chairs and table makes even the occupation of a jigsaw difficult. Curling up and sleeping in the day room is also frowned on, great attempt being made to underestimate the effects of drugs; the seven diabetics out of fifteen on one ward are attributed to the effects of Clozaril. Weight gains are tragic, sometimes six or more stone which requires new clothes in larger sizes. The means to commit suicide might have been reduced but the desire to die is greater than it ever was.

I can only believe that the Estates Manager was doing his utmost to cut down his maintenance expenditure by fitting very flimsy toilet seats which broke with the weight of anybody over nine stone sitting on them. One nurse became adamant that the girls were breaking them deliberately and we should do without any. She refused to put in chits for replacements. There was uproar and better quality seats were ultimately brought in. When the house was re-decorated in 2002 urinals, - seatless lavatories in mottled pink and pale mottled brown - were installed and it looked very much as though the intentions prevalent fifteen years earlier had manifested themselves again. The hateful mind that can insist on cold seatless lavatories for women is not fit to organise such a place. We were told the urinals were an American idea. With the reputation of American penal institutions I would not look to them for ideas of containment over here.

The visiting arrangements within a Sports Hall supposedly costing £25M but reputedly £100M, opened in the same year as the installations of urinals in 2002. Visitors sit on fixed chairs at low coffee tables so it is impossible to draw up one's chair to converse comfortably. Piped music is played softly to drown the voices of those at adjacent tables, which adds to the irritation. Refreshments are no longer served by patients acting as stewards; there is a vending machine. At least one prison has ripped out this arrangement and installed more acceptable furnishings but Broadmoor does not. The sports hall, multi gymnasium and 25-metre swimming pool are impressive but there is now more usage over the lunch hour and after work by staff than for patients during working hours. It is the same situation at Rampton where patients rarely visit the swimming pool.

Security increases constantly and by 2004 there were over two and a half thousand video cameras for four hundred patients; at any time fifteen staff are needed to be in the Radio Control room. This is more extreme security than is warranted by the average detainee but might yet be inadequate for an organised gang rescue attempt with helicopters, which has never happened as the detainees are rarely gangland connected. The few escapes have been made by exceptionally physically fit, agile, men, the resulting tightening of restrictions applying to the female wing too.

Jim Kay's escape involved sawing through the bars in dead of night and using sheet and bed cover as rope resulted in the female wing having its pretty, nursery-type bars replaced with plain unsawable steel, removal of room curtains, and bedclothes counted daily for the next five years despite the women being incapable of performing such a vanishing act. The lack of logic, which is accepted as normal and necessary by those in security, requires a lot of understanding. The men had their curtains replaced quite quickly and few male wards endured bed checks longer than eighteen months. Security needed to be tightened after a parole man, Roger Packham, attacked and raped a secretary in the Chaplain's Office. This was the second offence he had committed whilst in Broadmoor and it underlined how some men managed to get on in the system whilst non-rapists fared far worse.

The tinnitus started shortly after a couple of nurses smashed up my room ten years ago and said it was me. For this I was put on drugs and the ear buzzing started practically immediately. I would be on the medication still, shaking and hardly able to handwrite, but I took an overdose, spent forty-eight hours in an outside hospital, and the prescription stopped. A little nurse who was on duty at the time of the incident told me that there was nobody to whom she could report the incident. A few years later one of those nurses, while she slept soundly in the next room, lost her only son in an asthma attack so transferred to night duty until she retired. I was brought back to the present with a jolt. "They're doing phone calls", Mitch says.

A pay phone that takes cards has recently been installed on each ward and everyone is required to submit lists of those they intend phoning with the recipients signing their consent to accept the calls. The amount of paperwork involved in this exercise was astounding but Broadmoor, which could be said to run on military lines, never did things by halves. It was staggering how many relatives never wished to hear from their loved ones again and Broadmoor took precautions to see their wishes were adhered to. Tolerance all round seemed to be required. To suit staff tea break telephone calls were made after 6 p.m., sometimes the list of callers was so long that the nurse supervising the activity would intervene, "You can only have five minutes". At 14p a minute, later to rise to 25p, even with short phone calls many of us found our pocket money vanishing like puffs of air. There was often chaos with the allowable phone lists, particularly when the primitive computer system broke down and left off several pages so there was no record of who we could phone at all, but it was a breakthrough to be able to chat to my daughter and exchange news, not that I ever had much I wanted to impart but I loved hearing how the family were. It was reassuring.

I have a diary note for 6 October 1990. The UK joins the European RM on Monday – I doubt the users of the smoking day room know what that is or care a damn – and interest rates are reduced by 1% to 14%. Share prices rose. Something is happening somewhere but what happens in Broadmoor seems irrelevant to those outside. I sit in my room with the windows closed despite the central heating – the generator in the block next door is going full blast, the noise vibrates the windows and, weighing between either suffocating or going deaf, I opt to keep my hearing. There had been a public announcement that the woman who stole the Griffith's baby was being released after six months in Fairmile. What a change of policy. Another patient was sent here for such an offence; after ten years she was transferred to Fairmile where she married a patient and had a child of her own when she was sent back to Broadmoor, the baby taken into care. It was obvious that she was a changed person, far more mature than when she had been here previously. The memory of her caring husband holding her hand as she sobbed on visits that she wanted her baby, Claire, haunted me. Equality and fair play is in the mind of the administrators and their cruelty condoned. Few patients subjected to such traumas can see sense, let alone justice, in the minds of their keepers and can keep a cool head and rational view of the situation.

The Annual Show is the worst ever. Even Sheila gets a first for her thick shawl and Cathy a second for putting some dried flowers in a spoon. "How long did that take you", I say, "a day?". She grins. "No. Ten minutes". I had put in nothing as I was no longer in the Sewing Room but now working on the ward; in previous years I submitted pieces of crochet and so on. As the Show was in the Central Hall amongst the pillars painted gold and three shades of pink – which resembled *Ben Hur* rejects – visits were held in the sparse mini-hanger on the other side of the terrace, usually an occupational therapy area for difficult male patients. It was crowded for a Saturday morning – how sparse visitors were to become when they are banned from smoking and new rules recommended by Fallon and Tilt enforced. A male patient terminated his visit, he was crying; Liz terminated hers. "She was too hot", said the nurse.

My friend Heather is in fine form and we gurgle as each imitates the Social Worker. What is there about the Wiltshire accent that produces such mirth? "Listen to this logic, "says Heather, "I'll come tomorrow' he said and then when we'd finally fixed for next Friday he said he had to see the GP. If he'd come the next day he couldn't have made an appointment to see the GP so quickly. It's arranged now and the Probation Officer's coming too although it's not his workday. He has a job share and works three days a week. He comes in a pick-up. I think he's into pig farming".

As we walk back from the mini-hanger Chris, with feigned innocence, enquires, "Why do all the refreshments have to be taken back to the shop? Why can't they leave the coffee and everything till the afternoon?" Good question. Why cart a trolley full of eatables back and forth unnecessarily for a break of a couple of hours. "When I was in Holloway", I say, rising to the bait, "one of the prison officers had her wallet stolen from the staff canteen. I've never worked anywhere where that would happen". The escorts were horrified, "The staff you mean?" they cry.

On Saturday I take *The Times* and turn to the City page to do my sums to see how much I'm worth. I've not lost so much on the Stock Market this week as last. I'm like the fellow in the mental hospital who tells the doctor he's gaining weight. He lost 6 lbs. the previous week but only 4 lbs. this time. Broadmoor was co-operative in helping me participate in Maggy Thatcher's privatisations. It could take three weeks to sign a requisition and send out the relative cheque but share issues allowed five days; a Nursing Officer actually took one application form to the accounts department and licked down the envelope personally. Every little helps and it was one way of adding to the coffers.

I attend the Sewing Room, as relief from ward work, there is talk of Jeannette who has been in the Infirmary for a while and still shuffling badly with a spinal problem. "Dr Leven and Dr Horne say it's mental", says Shiela, "and they've upped her medicine a lot".
     "She had a blood test", said Dot.
     "Blood test won't reveal a back injury" I said, "Has she had an x-ray?". "No" was the answer. Not for the first time patients' views of medical treatment were in contrast to those of the doctors.

I found the handling of certain issues at Broadmoor rather difficult to accept. When a fifteen year old was admitted for cutting the brakes on her adopted mother's car and setting fire to their idyllic thatched cottage for being stopped going to a disco, the first activity the girl attended after arriving at Broadmoor was a disco. Discos at Broadmoor are slightly different from those outside where it is possible to meet unsuitable people but not as certain or obvious as meeting one or several at Broadmoor. This particular social was held in the mini-hanger as the Central Hall was out of action. I sat at the same table and noticed the girl giggling delightedly as she peered down the obligingly held open trousers of a serial rapist. They were both happy.

It was at one of these socials that I met Alan Reeve, whose escape to Holland created after waves. He told me that he had typed up the staff list, "There are nineteen Bonnetts", he said. Well, my Uncle Harry Davies family indulged in nepotism so I could not comment. Lack of numbers meant that women could attend twice as many social events than allowed the men. In the summer these were replaced by Sports Field and, once a month, chosen men visited the female wing for outside activities – usually sitting on the grass, the event being compulsory for the women so was regarded as a challenge to Women's Lib.

I also met Ahmed Alami who told me that the treatment he, a Jordanian, received living in Israel had brought him to this country to learn about paranoia from which he suffered; I understood he was undergoing analysis when he committed his terrible crime. He was also interested in the paranormal and we had several interesting discussions on this and related subjects. He told me that his father and brother were trying to arrange for him to be repatriated but I was unprepared for the announcement of it. The press and radio news all contained an item about the transfer to Israel of Dr Ahmed Alami whose father was the country's leading Arab; he was Mustapha of Jerusalem. I was appalled that such publicity should be afforded him, the Jews must be hugging themselves with delight and most of Broadmoor's psychiatrists were Jewish. Ahmed was taken back by Senior Nursing Officer Jerry Sharpe and psychiatrist Dr Boyce Lecouter, who both stayed in Israel a week. "It's necessary. They'd kill 'im," said Nurse Ron Attwood looking at me strangely; he told me the story of another man, taken back to Cairo, who was handed over and taken behind a hanger from which direction the Broadmoor staff heard the sound of a shot. Two senior nurses escorted a patient back to the West Indies. The patient, Audrey Pearce, was a nurse who had been in Broadmoor four years for hitting a policeman with her handbag when stopped in the street; she was released from her Barbados mental hospital the same day that she arrived. The escort staff stayed a week. There was some protest at the cost of taking patients back to their country of origin and, after the West Indian trip, it was said that a Mexican was actually driven to London Airport and put on a plane to return home unescorted. If released in the UK the man would have been subjected to "after-care" whether he required it or not.

Despite being well into October the heating is still off at school; the weather's non-seasonal and estimated to be 73°. There's a message that another friend and new baby daughter are visiting tomorrow; this was indeed a bonus, as messages are frequently not passed on. I was thus ready and waiting when the visit was called to find the baby had kept her parents awake since 4 a.m.; Mum and Grandma looked strained. I felt we were part of a club as I had been awake since midnight. I was shown photos of before, after and whilst the baby was delivered. I wonder how this generation will work out. It resents marriage, lives in what we called sin, and has illegitimate, now called love, children. The situation is puzzling, as clearly the grandmother is delighted with the new arrival, although she came from a class of people that would have hidden such a daughter away in an asylum about the time Broadmoor was built let alone acknowledge the grandchild. Mum retired to feed the baby - Nurse Hazel in attendance and I wondered what level of crude she had passed.

In 1987 *The Sunday Times* published an article of mine in their *Day In The Life* series. I had sent it in as a joke after reading Delia Smith's account of her day and I felt life in Broadmoor could be of interest. She got up, prayed, went for a walk, and prayed again. I was astounded when the editor wrote back asking me to make my piece longer. This time I thought the joke was on me but obliged with a paragraph on official visitors to Broadmoor and how it was possible to distinguish deer stalker hat magistrates from plastic bag carrying social workers and young policemen who came round in droves at least once a week, frequently more. What they came to see I have no idea but I conjectured what private company could be minus twenty-three (social workers from Hackney) of its personnel at any one time because they were on a trip to Broadmoor.

The response to the article was a surprise. A man in the salmon industry sent me half a smoked salmon – today that would not be allowed, no foodstuffs are permitted to be sent in – and there were a pile of letters. Two women told me their mothers had died in mental hospitals and both wondered how I had fared so long. Another was adamant that, in her parents' day in London's East End when the Krays ruled, it had been possible for old ladies to go out at night. The only person to get the postcode correct was a man in Washington DC who always affixed Langley stamps to imply he was CIA and sent me a photograph of a wall, the graffiti reading: "Pshrinks are quacks". Heather had responded by wanting to know how I could be got out. Fran had contacted me and asked if I would write her a play. She had an Arts Council grant that limited the production to no more than a monologue but I eventually wrote something – re-writes prior to computer access on my Silver Reed portable – and Fran added her ideas to it so that it did not look completely like my autobiography for fear of being sued. Fran's father was a lawyer. For the play, *The One-Sided* Wall Broadmoor had allowed the press (*Sunday Times, Evening Standard, Independent*, the tabloids kept away) to come onto the ward to interview me but had baulked at the BBC's *Women's Hour* bringing in their recording equipment, the BBC could come in but not record me which was typical of the attitude of Broadmoor. The reviews were for the show at the Bush Theatre were good, John Mortimer writing that it would be deplorable if the story the play told was true which it was. Cindy Oswin was the star, she didn't look like me but that was irrelevant. I naturally thought the *Sunday Times* article and the play would speed my discharge but the powers-that-be dug their heels in and I was largely ignored. Broadmoor allowed the play in and I was amazed how many patients and staff turned up to see it; I had objected when I heard patients were to be charged and my protest was listened to. The show was free. Methuen published it in their series *Plays By Women: 8* but all this was in the past. The producer had now found a partner, started a family, and the theatre no longer in her equation but we always had plenty to chat about. Her baby was adorable.

When I returned to the ward I was told I had a box. In it was a box of Cadbury's Dairy Milk. A couple of minutes later the Sister in charge called me to the office, "Janet", she says all friendly smiles, "tell me the gossip, when's it going to rain?" Oh Hu. "No gossip", I say, "I've been cuddling a month-old baby all afternoon". Sister's face dropped. She didn't want to talk babies. She wanted a chocolate. She wouldn't let me escape easily.

"Jimmy Savile", she said, "have you got him a girl friend yet?" Why me? Jimmy was nearly a fixture at Broadmoor, appearing at fete days and organising pop groups for socials. For some years he had a flat at Broadmoor.

"Oh. He can do his own running", I said, "he's got his secretary over there. Say. Does John come from Minnesota or Manitoba?"

"John?" Sister has lost the thread.

"Nurse John. My Primary Nurse. He told me he was American, too short for the British police so joined the army, went to Australia and joined the South African Police."

"John", she said looking through the window, "told me he lived in Leicester". The appearance of Anne, on of the OT staff ended the inane interview.

94

I woke up unable to move. I was in agony. My back had gone. The duties of ward worker for £25 a month with best room involved doing the ward washing twice a week when the residents put out their dirty clothes to be stuffed into the washing machine and tumble dryer, clearing up and cleaning the kitchen and dining room, washing up (again in a machine) and carrying heavy food boxes downstairs after the meals were over. Later on the porters would be instructed to carry the boxes, they refused; then the kitchen workers had to carry them; an internal lift was eventually built at easily a quarter of a million pounds so that the boxes were hoisted up and wheeled onto the wards. The process of reaching the point where the lifts were actually installed took years the aggro and tension en route unimaginable. We were still at the stage of getting female patients to lift male loads.

I partnered Ma, a trans-sexual who was weak by male standards but strong by female ones and she had been sweetness itself taking the heavier loads and helping me out, so I did most of the laundry. A system of carrying by all members of the ward could have been instituted to spread the load around but staff maintained this breached security which I interpreted as they didn't want to organise it. I was threatened with being sent to the Medical Centre to recover – a ghastly experience – but managed to persuade the Sister to leave me lying flat for another day, I hoped the muscles would drift back into alignment by then. This had happened before, a couple of years previously, and I'd slept flat without pillows ever since; I was lucky then. I was this time but clearly I should not do the lifting. I did not want to lose my room and get relegated back to the dormitory – later to be closed – or to a titchy cell called room.

We now had a charge nurse who had come from the male side with an awful reputation of threatening behaviour with removal of room and banishment to dormitory for the slightest deviation although so far he had not displayed symptoms of his reputation one did not know which way things would go. He was ultimately to leave under a cloud after being videoed slashing tyres in a supermarket's invalid car park. The story was that he was angry that his daughter had been unable to find a parking space for her invalid carriage so he took the law into his own hands. His supporters maintained he was suffering from nervous strain from work on this ward thereby publicising how terrible the patients were on York II, now called Leeds Ward. The attempts of Chief Executive Alan Franey to humanise the institution had included using names for wards instead of numbers. All the houses were called after counties and the wards after towns or cities. Thus York House now had Harrogate, Leeds and Sheffield instead of York I, II and III. I did wonder at Somerset House calling one of their wards Mendip and if those who christened the female wing houses York and Lancs had the Wars of the Roses in mind.

As no alternative to the ward work was offered I carried on with off duty days in the sewing room. This situation was perhaps typical of many where staff were unable to deal with a matter. As we stand in the medicine queue before tea Sue is called in to see Dr Horne who tells her that the trip to see her grandmother in a geriatric hospital on Tuesday (with two male staff, handcuffs and one female) is off as she is high security and shouldn't know in advance that she's going out. She screamed, "Oh for f…. " etc and was put into seclusion; noises including, "'Ow can I move when you're sitting on my 'ead" reverberate down the corridor.   It's all very well altering appointments but if Sue's grandmother was expecting her she would be upset too.

After tea, very late, we spot there's a notice on the board reading, "Prison Officers Association are taking industrial action on the 13th when no visits will be allowed". The notice has materialised too late for Sal's visitors to be contacted and they will be turned away after a long journey.   I put my head in the office to say to Nurses Colleen and Vicky, "That's mean". "We don't think so", they said.   If "they" are all in it, this accounts for my recent broken nights' sleep.

On the face of it night inspection was part of the care routine but it entailed flashing a torch through the window at the bottom of the door whilst looking through the spy hole, which some staff were not sufficiently agile or tall enough for this to constitute a comfortable operation. Most staff merely flashed the torch in the room and moved on to the next room, the amount of time they spent looking could not have revealed much. Beds were required to be situated in front of the door, in line with the window so staff could see the patient.   Correctly the torches' aim was for the sleeper's shoulders, if they moved, intimating breathing, the patient was all right.   Frequently the bulb would be too bright and nobody was around to change it for one more suitable for night inspection. If the light flashed across the face the sleeper would inevitably stir if not waken.   Patients who snored fared better as they could be heard to be alive.   I frequently lay awake and counted when the staff came round, some were more vigilant than others whose rounds were infrequent, and I often found it difficult to go back to sleep once I had been woken. The female wing was short of electricity so, although permitted on the male side, personal televisions were not allowed on the female side until the late 80's when power points were installed in the rooms, so radios were battery operated which was expensive. If one was woken in the night there was nothing one could do except lie there. There was no getting up to have a drink and a pee and going back to bed again. Flashing torches across the faces of sleepers and switching on lights in the middle of the night is usually a herald of unrest; at the best of times it could be called counter-productive practice but one that is difficult to change, management must cover themselves "if anything happens". It also ensures that night staff have something to do and do not go to sleep on duty. Many is the time that I have thought of committing suicide after being woken to see I was all right but common sense told me that the reason for my death would be denied, I could imagine it being attributed to my mental state. "We're doing our job" would cry the staff when they were challenged.

This provocative method of care was perhaps typical of so much in the psychiatric system which required of itself to show that something was being done when in fact that something was superfluous and counter to the patient's interests. A similar situation existed with social workers whose role had become little more than compiling reports for tribunals for which they were required to visit relatives who did not always at first appreciate that no help would be forthcoming, the object of the visit was merely to collect information for tribunal reports and case conferences. Where there was family conflict the social worker felt vilified.

I've endured staff industrial action at increased rents, for more pay, greater staff levels.... One action was still talked about although it had happened sixteen years previously, before I arrived, when staff had refused to dispense injections so the doctors had to do them and there had been no post and no visits. On one occasion the Sister called us to the day room and announced that staff would work to rule and there would be "no movement of patients" which meant no work or activities. "That's not 'work to rule', which is what railway workers do", I said, "They work to the rules to make them ridiculous. You aren't doing that. You are making your own rules and not working at all", Sister was furious but everyone laughed and from thereon the term "industrial action" was used for such occurrences, still an inaccurate term, there being little industry on the wards where the trouble lay. What is it this time?

The fire alarm goes off at 7.30 p.m. and we troop out into the dark. We do not doubt it's Lizzie again, on the ward downstairs, because her visit's off due to the "action". After the alarm and we're all back in her friend Vera sits sobbing on the floor in a corner of the day room. "They part us. They don't part the f... others", she wails. "Lizzie and I looked after each other. She wants to come back up". Oh dear. I can't tell her Lizzie's husband objects to the company she keeps and does not want his wife dominated by Vera. Later her friend says the staff say there really was a small fire, cause unknown, "They're probably telling me that so I don't nag at Lizzie", she sobs again refusing to believe anything she is told. It was probably burnt toast setting off the alarm.

Staff say the "No Visits Industrial Action" is because of the budget. Broadmoor is like the prodigal son, a spendthrift playing up for more. One Sports Day had cost £3K; the teams from each house had been equipped with special outfits and there were lots of prizes from the stalls. I had returned to the ward carrying a box of them including musical jewellery case, boxes of chocolates…. Few were unaware that this was compensation for overcrowded conditions and staff had endeavoured to be kind but when for years we managed with one small washing machine on a ward for thirty eight the generosity in one direction was overweight.

There were now cutbacks….. A nurse states that our shoe issue was unnecessary; I believe that this was the last time a lorry from Staffordshire came loaded with shoes for the female wing. It was always badly organised; those in first could purchase extra pairs with their own money which left insufficient pairs for the ones going in last to even draw their issue. *There were usually cries of disappointment from the last in and on one occasion a woman was sent to the Block where she stayed for the next five years. All because there were no shoes in her size and she protested.* One year there were a load of fur-lined boots on offer – a strange choice for the over-heating of Broadmoor but they were attractive – and the selected favoured ones allowed first buy. I had wondered if these low-priced goodies were off the back of a lorry and everybody laughed when I said Broadmoor would be the last place the police would look for them. One year I acquired a good pair of hand-made leather-lined walking shoes, "Made In Poland" which lasted me for years until I had them mended and they became waterproof no longer.

A card from Hereford. The social worker's visit went OK. He had told my friend that the ridiculous case conference stemmed from my complaint to the Mental Health Commissioners. I wonder. From where I stand those in authority have no desire to accept responsibility so involve others in the hope that somebody will take me, and others, off their hands. My sleep is fretful. The central heating is on, the pipes gurgle all night and the tension emanating from staff over their action is disturbing. From experience of no movements on the wards for a month and being told that, prior to my admittance, the staff had stopped both post and visits, we gauged that there had been some embargo to prevent things going so far again but what was available would be rigorously enforced. What will they think up next? Strange how more pay and higher staff ratio can enable the inmates to sleep better. Some cannot stand the strain and hefty 5'8" Jeannette attacks 84-year old 5'0" Lily in the dormitory. There's no justification for it but it adds to the tension building up because of the "industrial action"; the more incidents there are will substantiate staff claims that theirs is a dangerous occupation and they need more staff, more money. I wonder if the rise in the number of fits by epileptic patients is recorded and analysed, they are usually the ones to react the most and since being here I have learnt to use them like barometers to gauge the atmosphere. I feel jaded through broken sleep, some days hardly knowing what day it is, like old Margaret is permanently, but time passes quickly enough and remains in the memory with cameo sketches. Arthur Koestler, one-time science correspondent to the *Daily Telegraph,* as well as claiming that communism, Catholicism and psychiatry were all instruments of revolution, also maintained that times of greatest social upheaval stemmed from sun spots. Whatever it is that stirs trade unions into activity I cannot attribute to sunny connexions, even spots. It's just money. Money and nothing else but perhaps the sun spots provoke them more. Dr Cyril Levin with whom I raised the subject of sun spots and mental illness pooh-poohed the idea as nonsense. Puffing away at his dog end he stoutly refuted that meteorological events affected people in any way whatever. I dare not ask him if he had a headache prior to a thunderstorm and kept quiet that I did.

In the salon one of the hairdressers says she's been to a Marks & Spencers customer account Christmas Show and was delighted when I remarked, "Just like for the Queen at Harrods". I can cut my own hair but the ward scissors are, in the interests of security, blunt. So for a small sum and a break from the ward I have a trim and blow dry with qualified coiffeurs.

Fran, the baby and father visited again which was lovely. They all looked so well and the baby had grown 10cms and looked far more in proportion – perfect. A part-time psycho-analyst, Dr Murray Cox, (4 hours a week @ £25p.h. in 1977) was patron of the Royal Shakespeare Company (RSC); with the interest of Mark Rylance the actor, later the obvious choice to be director of The Globe Theatre, brought in several plays, *Hamlet, Romeo and Juliet, King Lear,* and Thomas Heywood's *A Woman Killed with Kindness* which, although a near contemporary of William Shakespeare, was written in far more comprehensible English than the Bard of Stratford with his flowery prose. I went only to *Hamlet* and the Heywood production but will always remember Mark Rylance as Hamlet paddling across the Central Hall in a bathtub.

There were a couple of snags to these memorable productions, performed in the round, some of the audience sitting on stage, the cast in modern dress. At the workshop held after the performance inmates were expected to say things like, "I felt like that when I killed my father-in-law". Then there was the other handicap of the Central Hall being too small to accommodate everyone who wanted to attend. Not just nursing staff wanted to go but teachers, secretaries, you name it. When Sister Irene called me into the office to enquire if I had forgotten to put my name down for the Wilde Company's *Measure for Measure,* I replied, "No. I hadn't forgotten. It's just that last time the hall was so hot and crowded my tinnitus made sitting there agony".

At school the tutor is appalled when I say that John Major's nil rates inflation scheme is under way. "Nil." He exclaims in horror, "We've a pay claim in and are 15% down already". "It hasn't a snowball's chance", I console him, "but the clothing manufacturers are co-operating. The Clothes Show on Sunday's TV showed the cost of women's clothing must go down, the latest short tube dresses use minimal material". I was reminded of the theory that when hemlines rise so does the Stock Market.

The ward buzzes with a news item in the *Daily Express.* There has been a disciplinary hearing by the nursing profession and three nurses from Broadmoor have been accused of unprofessional conduct. We are amazed. We can all recall some shocking occasions; my own memory includes a ward sister with an obsession over a crippled woman with one lung who claimed her crippledom was caused by nurses at Rampton injecting into the sciatic nerve and was in process of suing them; Broadmoor had done its best to convince her she had had childhood poliomyelitis. After several days of extreme harassment the Sister put the patient in the garden one chilly October day in only her nightclothes; the girl, Gwendolyn Hargreaves, had recounted her experiences to me - at one point the ward were marshalled into the garden where we could hear Gwen's screams as she was being held under bath water by a group of staff and she said she had been forced to take some concoction that had caused her uncontrollable diarrhoea which the staff had jeered at. Because I knew what was happening I was banished to the Block for fifteen months without an incident on my part. Gwen was sent back to Rampton where she died six months' later. "You're not wanted on the ward," the MO had told me. "Sorry you're not doing well", had said the psychiatrist knocking his pipe on the side of the desk. On the Block I saw male nurses in the female bathroom, "It's our job", they would say gazing at the naked bodies; one threw a young girl against a room wall; two nurses who smashed up my room said it was me who had done it, several patients were left for days with no pot, food or water or clothes – most people could tell a tale or two. MIND stated that a third of the staff were unfit to work on the wards and some other organisation had stated it needed only 2% of a workforce to cause disruption.

The three nurses highlighted in the *Express* had done no more than what we regarded as normal. Nurses Karen Woods, Julie Thompson and Linda Lleung had been accused of singing, "Here we go, here we go", the football song, when dishing out medicines, and telling a patient who complained at the noise, "You've got voices". Julie Thompson is said to have thrown water in a patient's face. The news item was headed: "Three nurses at Broadmoor accused of 'beating patient'". The nurse bringing the complaint, Crawley, now a sister in another hospital, states she falsified the incident report, as she was frightened of the other nurses. She's not the only frightened person. I reckoned management staff kept their tyres from being slashed with their offhand replies to patients' serious allegations. I recalled the demand for an enquiry that never happened into the death of an attractive twenty-one year old, Liz Finch, by her father, a major in the British Army. "She choked on her vomit," read the coroner's report, which gave no indication of the trauma she was undergoing after being demoted with little or no cause to the Block. The demotion had stemmed from staff intolerance and the need to make more space for a new admittance. Another frequent cause of death was "cardiac arrest" though we all die of that. I had become used to verbal abuse and had never complained of it, it was the more physical aspects that formed the basis of my dissidence. Another surprise was that such hearings are open to the public; I would have thought they would be held in camera.

I didn't think much of the video the younger members of the ward (now universally called "young thugs" or "the gang") were watching so I decide to do my ironing. Both iron and board are kept locked up but available on application. Ma has got there first and was busy in the corridor; I stay and chat while she finishes. "How did you get on?" I knew she had seen a doctor today which generally heralds a tribunal or possible transfer to another mental hospital. "Oh. The doctor you mean. He wasn't a psychiatrist. Dr

Horne called him in.   The questions he asked…. I've lost a lot of weight".

"How much?"

"I was eleven twelve and I'm now eight stone".

"In how long?" I had seen her looking ill but hadn't realised how serious it could be.   "A month" she replied, "he took a finger prick sample and I'm to have another blood test next week. He thinks it's cancer".

"A friend of mine lost a lot of weight", I said, "she had one diagnosis after another with diets to match. Ultimately she settled on Crohns Disease. I hope they find what it is, it's worse if they can't find anything and guessing is hell". As I walked off I assumed it couldn't be AIDS, Ma's been here too long. Next day Nurse John is adamant that Ma does not have AIDS.

"The staff've been asking me who I've mucked about with in 'ere", Mitch says later, "but in fact lesbians are the least risk section of the community provided they're not drug addicts or haemophiliacs".

"The ward's a can of worms", I say.

The gang watch videos, three of them, all day; those wanting any other programme, *Blind Date* or the *News* for instance, have to retreat to the smoking room whether they smoke or not. The gang have taken over the ward; when others watch anything the gang do not want their screams of chatter, passing of wind and accompanied wild laughter, drive even the brave to seek refuge elsewhere. It was impossible to watch the Remembrance Service so I retire to my room and type out a piece of fiction, the story line reflecting my sorrow at the lack of respect by a section of the younger generation.

106

As I wait downstairs to go to the Education Centre, Alvada rushes up to me. She is a ghastly grey. "Did you know Joan's dead? She died in her sleep last night" she said, the pallor of her face almost reflecting that of her hair. I didn't know. Joan had had a couple of heart attacks and I assumed she had had another one. I was sad but it happens. She was, what, sixty five. It's usual when somebody dies for the ward to be gathered together and a formal announcement made to stop conjecture. Perhaps somebody had forgotten to tell us. At lunch time Ma tells me she heard Joan "hung herself". In the afternoon I go to the library where Alvada looks blank-eyed and Margaret is ashen. Shiela says, "It's been on the radio" and "treated as suicide". Later Nurse V tells me that it was the duty doctor's first suicide and he's still shaking this morning; he's only been here two months. Then she said, "Joan was found with a Bible in her hand". I felt physically sick and blamed myself for chatting only with Alvada when I went downstairs for a visit a few evenings before; I had merely nodded to Joan as she passed and said, "Hi", conscious that Alvada would get fidgety if I conversed with anybody but her. I'd been fond of Joan who was a quiet soul, she was very kind and helpful, from mending garments to lending knitting needles; she had maimed her young son in response to voices in her head thirty-five years previously and defeated the maxim that penitence be a requirement for release. She was penitent eternally. She would have done anything to undo what she had done and she paid the penalty for it. Her first five years in Broadmoor were spent in Intensive Care, the Block, tormented, wracked, by guilt and drugged to the hilt, others swanned through saying "I'm sorry" at intervals for record in the files and fared far better. Whilst otherwise perfectly sane and sensible, Joan had one trait; she refused to admit that her husband had divorced her to marry a housekeeper for their two children and she maintained that he would one day come and get her out of Broadmoor. Till she died, Joan's husband was loyal and faithful to her in her imagination. I knew she had expressed the wish to go and live with Dora, an ex patient who kept an animal sanctuary but the ward psychiatrist, Dr Chandra Ghosh, refused to countenance such a proposition and had suggested transfer to another mental hospital. Such suggestions always produced more voices of her husband from Joan but whether these were real or she knew their manufacture would stop the transfer I have no idea. The suggestion had recently been raised again. I blamed myself for not talking to her but my elevation to ward work had reduced the opportunity to meet her in the Sewing Room where she was a mainstay.

My Hereford friend visited. It was a relief to see someone from outside, the atmosphere on the wards is over-subdued and oppressive but she clearly was upset when I said that the delay in doing anything constructive from the tribunal boded ill. Not for the first time she dissolved into tears when I said I would be surprised if I were released as those in authority had tried to kill me on arrest and the lies to get me committed to Broadmoor were very difficult to contradict. She blanched when I reminded her that the tribunal report had stated on the first page, "To be detained through reason of mental illness", the illness unspecified; page two stated that I should be got out quickly through reason of age and suggested I live with her in Hereford. Back on the ward I am told, "John King has been waiting to see you since two". Visiting is two till four. It is now ten past four. John

King materialised as John Waters who had been earlier, gone away and returned.

"I realise I don't know Janet Cresswell", he starts, "and if I'm to back her release I must know more about her".   Why can't he use direct speech instead of this third person nonsense?

"I thought we'd got past that point", I said and he explained that SHSA would come back with questions.

"Why don't you wait and see what they ask or ask them in advance?" I say, "instead of guessing what they want to know" but I was aghast that he wanted me to "exercise your legal right" and put in for yet another tribunal. I had just had one and that was endurance. This meant somebody didn't like the last tribunal result, was blocking it and would try to get what they wanted at the next one.   It didn't matter what I did.   Any tribunal I put in for would be met by a larger and more powerful team than the one I had.   I was spared further harassment as Nurse Irene came to break us up for tea; John Waters said he'd see me again next week and I told Sister Irene that he needed some happy pills; his gloom was catching.

Most of us sign a bulk requisition form for flowers for Joan, the funeral will be in the Chapel here on Tuesday afternoon, the inference being that she will be buried in Broadmoor's cemetery. I feel sick. I am deeply upset and feel that this is her family's final rejection.   Can't her two brothers, who took turns to visit her once a month over the past thirty five years, afford a cremation? Or did she want this?   I doubt it. Julie, who knows everything, informs us that tolls have to be paid if bodies are taken over county borders. It sounds medieval. The feeling of disgust persists.   I hope I have the wrong end of the stick. One of the

Sewing Room staff maintains that Joan "often rattled on" about the *Thirty Nine Steps* and Ariadne's thread but I could not recall her mentioning it to me. "Apart from that", Nurse Tilly said, "she was fine".

Veronica is back on the ward. We all know to be careful what we leave around and to guard our washing in the laundry room; she is prone to select items she fancies, wait till the ward can't stand her any more and move her to another where she will sell the items to the inmates there. There was an arrangement whereby three wards took it in six-week stints to have her. On the subject of Veronica both patients and staff are unanimous in agreement. If anything is required to get a pay dispute settled by causing unrest, it's having Veronica on the ward. Mitch is locked in but whether the event is related to Veronica I know not.

The gang again play videos all day despite "the tracking's not working" and a ward meeting. As usual we were told all the things the staff found irritating in us, "You must come promptly for medicines", "You must not push the chairs together to go to sleep in the day room" etc. but there was little time for our complaints. I wandered into the smoking room and saw the Robert Powell version of *The Thirty Nine Steps* was showing. I paid little attention until the book is retrieved from the Post Office and hear the words, "The Thirty nine steps and Ariadne's thread". Oh no. My thought went back to Joan. Did she feel that she laid the foundation for her husband to escape the labyrinth? I am interrupted by Nurse Jan who enquires if I am going to the funeral service, which is the same day as the Tory leadership vote. "I don't think I can bear to", I said, "I don't feel I could contain myself from

confronting her brothers about letting her be buried
here. By attending the service I would condone the
arrangements."   The Vicar's wife tries to console me,
"It's a beautiful spot", she says, "just outside the walls"
where the graves were unmarked for fear of vandalism
– from sane people outside – but a record of burials
meticulously recorded.

"Medicines" are called. This is a hallowed ritual
that nothing must intrude. Even those not on
medication have to sit in the non-smoking day room,
which must be silent, radio and television off.   How
many unfinished films have I watched in here because
the switch is turned off at a climatic point?   Inmates
leave the day room, walk along the corridor to the
medicine hatch in alphabetical order.   They need to
know who is in front of them so wrath is not incurred
by holding up the line. Several wear their Walkman's,
emit buzzy noises to those around, go into a coma and
cannot hear when they are shouted at. I knew a man
once who, with a surname starting with 'W', seriously
considered changing his name to one starting with 'A'
so he could head the distribution list. Nobody at
Broadmoor changed their name for that reason; the
entire ward had to wait in silence to the bitter end until
the medicine ritual was finished.   Toilet and washroom
doors are locked to prevent those who want to spit the
stuff out spitting, officially described as "a safety
precaution to save lives".   Most I know never found
difficulty secreting unwanted medication despite the
locked doors.

On Tuesday I go to the hairdressers but don't go back
to the Sewing Room afterwards. This is a change
from the determination to get rid of us and have the
ward empty as was the staff policy of a couple of years
back. Mitch is out of seclusion and pales at thought of

111

Joan being buried here. She had reported Joan to a ward sister who had left and died at least six years previously for berating Mitch at a mealtime on the subject of John Buchan's classic novel *The Thirty Nine Steps*". (Not again!). Mitch had been too busy eating to listen fully to what Joan said but the Sister had been adamant, "It's all in her head. It's nonsense" – typical of a professional diagnosis. Mitch adds, "Bet they've saved on a shroud and bury her in a seclusion gown".

"You can wrap my ashes in an overtime sheet", remarks Nurse John.

The news on TV is all pictures of Big Ben – without Richard Hannay hanging on to stop the hands moving. Michael Heseltine has challenged Margaret Thatcher for leadership; if she goes down the Tory Party will face a complete decline just as Labour did when Harold Wilson resigned. I realise for the first time that Gorbachev in Russia, George Bush (the first) in the USA and Mitterrand in France are all having their leaderships challenged. Strange how world leaders are toppled so easily while their subjects in middle-management at Broadmoor stay put despite results. *The Telegraph* wonders where they will all be next year. I wonder where we will be. I conjecture on the Russian revolution, which caused such pain and havoc but left the legal profession and penal system intact.

Party politics affect places like this. Most mental hospitals and prisons were in disarray, riot state, at the end of the Wilson era through overcrowding and over control so the first thing the Thatcher Government did in 1979 was try to reduce the numbers of those detained. The ward I am on now housed thirty-eight women in 1976, the number is down to twenty eight and will become fourteen and less by the year 2000 when most ward managers will have a secretary whilst the Head of Psychology will not. Another strange fact was that Margaret Norris, a member of the psychology team, had conducted a survey into discharged patients to discover that most had abandoned taking their medication without apparent adverse effect; any failure rate was mainly attributed to alcohol. It seemed very odd that such research could be carried out but the findings not acted upon in Broadmoor where forced drugging caused so much distress and problem.

When I first came it took me a while to understand why a nurse sat outside the bathroom door with a book calling names, often at an inconvenient moment, berating those who did not answer the call promptly and ticking off those who had a bath. It was not that the women required this regimentation; it was that two baths and shortage of time available on the wards necessitated a strict regime so everyone could stay clean. The shower over the bath was unusable – very long cold leg of water and then scalding hot, impossible to regulate. The baths had detachable taps that had to be handed in when the bather had finished and were kept in a locked cupboard when not in use. A major search was instigated when one tap went missing. It was found in the OT waste bin, which no patient could have reached. Another instance of staff behaviour. Whilst the rest of the country was reduced to a meagre water allowance because of the 1977 hot summer and drought, Broadmoor enjoyed all the water it could use. "We have our own reservoir", 'they' would say.

The domestic washing machine, totally inadequate for thirty-eight women was joined by a big industrial one after a ward sister asked me to write to Jimmy Savile for help on the matter. Lower numbers was a relief. Thirty- eight to one small washing machine was a nightmare.

I was the only female going to the Education Centre that afternoon; as I am escorted there I see the hearse drawn up outside the Chapel entrance and I ask Escort Shirley if I can look at the flowers the girls have contributed. I was looking at some large chrysanthemums and two bunches of freesias where the coffin had lain and trying to read the tags as visitors swept by. I recognised one of Joan's brothers, who looked very white and drawn, and his wife. I hop back sharply to avoid being noticed and go into school. Iris told me later that she had gone and it was a very moving service with people in tears and lots of flowers. I said nothing about the funeral to the Vicar's wife who teaches in the school when I saw her next day.

The social worker sees me with "How is Janet?", instead of "How are you?" When I addressed him as "you" he lent back in his chair and said, "Oh not 'you'". I find communication with him a great strain and walk out. I really cannot understand what he needs. I refuse to believe that he does not know either.

My Hereford friend visits and we conjecture what the Queen has said to Maggie and vice versa. We have a patient on the ward whose sisters cooked dinner parties for Prince Charles and she says the Queen dislikes Margaret Thatcher. I maintain that Maggie had told ER it was time she retired. I am convinced she was instrumental in getting Prince Charles to marry. We are waited on by David C, who brings our tea. He says he's been out with the Vicar to Windsor to a convent. "I taught a nun Braille", he says. "I once knew a fellow who claimed to be the only Jew in a monastery but this is the first time I've met a man who's been in a nunnery", I joke as I signed the chit to be debited to my account. Visitors were allowed into the canteen and I purchased a couple of yoghurts and signed another chit to be debited for these.

Broadmoor can be criticised for petty mindedness but attention to details included meticulously itemising all purchases on a statement received by each patient each month provided the computer did not break down. Being able to pay for tea assuaged some way the feeling of helplessness I experienced at the generosity of those who braved searching and the onerous reception to visit me – they even had to tip out any pills they carried before being allowed in. I do not doubt that getting in to visit at Broadmoor was a topic of conversation to liven pub or after dinner. By 2003 one friend told me it was easier to visit somebody on California's Death Row than Broadmoor but once in, even the horrid new visiting arrangements were superior.

John Major is now Prime Minister. He reminds me in appearance of my father. A grey man in a dark grey suit. I would always describe my father as well-intentioned but fuddy-duddy although at fancy dress parties he could appear as Mahatma Gandhi. John Major, despite his circus upbringing, is rather similar but much richer.

Several of us come to the conclusion that the ward is run by those speaking Widling English; all three ward heads are now either Welsh or West Indian but that is not the reason I spend the morning on the ward to see the Mental Health Commissioners. Whilst waiting I hear the latest ward psychiatrist, Fiona Mason, reply to an elderly solicitor's, "Presumably because the Home Secretary wouldn't accept it" with "Oh. The Home Secretary has agreed it". What can that be about? I wonder if the Home Secretary has even been shown what he's agreeing to and how much the Parliamentary Under-Secretary's are responsible for. At my tribunal the solicitor said privately that David Mellor's desk at the Home Office was piled high with unsigned papers. Dr Chandra Ghosh has told me that, although she is being moved to the male side she is still keeping those women patients whose cases are in process and she is handling personally. I am one of them. I guess she is going to the male side to get things moving over there. What a travesty of justice this system is where people cannot be released because of the ineptitude of those in charge.

From the Canteen sale I buy a doll for my grand-daughter. It reminds me of Gelsemina, an Italian doll my mother bought for my daughter when she was a little girl and now grown up with her own family. On sight of it my grand-daughter calls her new doll Alice. I had lots of dolls when I was a child; the best ones were made in Germany. I remember breaking one but my upbringing with Nathanial Hawthorne's *Tanglewood Tales* persuaded me that by planting the pieces in a flower bed new dolls would grow like soldiers emerged from the ground from planted shields. My mother did not understand at all.

Visits are cancelled for tomorrow (6 December) due to "industrial action", a strange term for non-activity. "No movement" so no work areas or functions either.

Mitch conjectures whether Veronica will get her teeth from the dentist.

Veronica did get her teeth. A previous dentist, a Mr McVerry, had refused to fit her with any as he said she couldn't manage them; here she is with a full set and, incredibly, no problems with them. I remember one woman emerging from his surgery and the nurse enquiring, "All right dear?"

"I don't know", said Barbara in a strong Birmingham accent, "he stuck the injection down 'ere and filled one up there". The present dentist is quite different. His breath does not smell; he is polite and very gentle. When it is not possible for the ward to supply an escort to get the patient to the Medical Centre and the patient's requirements can be met on the ward, the dentist will come over to the ward. He even extracted a tooth this way.

We spend the "holiday" created by the industrial action with Christmas decoration activity. There is a prize for the best decorated ward and this, understandably, depends more on the staff participating than on the patients' contribution.

While the "action" continues it materialises that OT staff have been given a pep talk not to sit on their backsides despite having no patients and certainly the sewing room staff had shown initiative and stuck up some tinsel bits. "What did you do after that?" someone enquired and received a gleam in the eye from them. We can guess…….

A week later the "industrial action" was off then on again. "Something must have happened", everyone thought the non-event was off. This lack of communication is something to which everybody becomes inured. There were no visits that day or the next day either. Sister Sue gets social worker John to phone Fran to stop her coming. I read *The Times* item on the action to the occupants of the full staff room. "It isn't true", they cry, "We've not been locked out by management". Later we have a choice of two packets of sweets or some fags, "Present from Management", we are told and assume this is compensation for no visits and being confined to the wards. Julie, ever on the ball, arranges a thank you note for these and asks for a new record player and video. I refuse to sign. "It sticks in my gullet", I say. It snows nearly all day so maybe it's just as well visits are cancelled, the roads are treacherous. To prove it, all trains from Euston are cancelled.

News that the release of the Guildford Six has been deferred till after Christmas has shocked *The Times* and I can think of more to shock them... me for instance. Dr Ghosh has depressed me with an interview intimating that nothing is moving on my behalf. I'm cheered up again by a visit from Fran and the baby with my friend from Hereford even though it's in the less comfortable mini-hanger. I say this for my friends; they do not take intimidation lightly. They visit when they can despite obstacles like not knowing if they will be let in. They are British and brought up to be stoic through thick and thin although the thick that invents the criteria takes some accounting.

The music centre is on in the day room most medicine times. This is a break-through for some who like the choice of sound preferred by members of the gang. For others it is irritating. For some, other people's noise is like the smell of other people's oranges but

one must not knock overtures of rules' relaxation.
There is talk of abolishing uniforms.   Unthinkable.
Are staff now to be given clothing allowance for having
to provide their own clothing?   What will the Tailors'
Shop and Sewing Room do without altering staff
uniforms?   Staff dresses arrive with unstitched hems
to cater for the long and the tall; the hem measuring
was carried out by Sewing Room staff and the patients
stitched; there was a stack of obsolete dresses as the
design and shade of colour was changed regularly,
each change requiring each nurse to have a statutory
six dresses in a range of uninspiring colours – mainly
blue, pink or green with a splattering of mud brown -
which we used for rags and other purposes.

One of the other ways of using discarded uniforms and
other clothing was making bunting for Sports Day.   It
decorated the field and acted as markers for the races.
A Social Worker, Dougie Hunter, had "loaned"
Broadmoor's bunting for an event in Crowthorne for
the Silver Jubilee; it had not been returned and Duggy
had put in a request for the Sewing Room to
manufacture a mile of little flags for the coming year.
After we had been at it ten days, me and others cutting
triangles to the point we had sore hands from gripping
the scissors, others machining onto enormous rolls of
tape, I costed the project.   At a minimum of £3 a dress
and discarded nightdresses etc. we had so far cut up
£1200 of brand new material.   I recited this at lunch,
the ward Sister Jane heard me and presented herself
in the Sewing Room that afternoon.   The project was
finished. We had done enough.

When I arrived, the social worker, Duggy Hunter had
offered to arrange collection of my goods and chattels
from my flat but it never happened. Months elapsed

with his, "Let me have a list" and me replying, "I've sent you one", and sending him another until the point was reached when I was informed by a friend that my flat had been vandalised and left in ruins. There was nothing left. I was lucky to sell the property and under escort was allowed to visit my bank to collect the deeds to hand over to my solicitor and visit the flat. Dougie came too in another car. The stench as the door was opened, the smashed remains of what had been built-in cupboards were piled in every room; no carpets were left, even the kitchen and bathroom sinks had been taken. I had difficulty not picking up a piece of wood and hitting Dougie with it; we had to eat our packed lunch sitting in the vehicle on Hampstead Heath, my flat was not habitable for even that much. I had been allowed to buy cakes for the ward from the Continental cake shop near the bank and the girls were delighted at sight of the two giant-sized gateaux I took back for them. I was nonplussed, however, at being thanked for a piece by a member of staff from another ward, I thought I had brought back enough for two days, not feed the entire female wing staff. All in all I did not thank Dougie Hunter for anything and it was some time before I recovered from the experience of the vandalising and lack of police ability to catch anybody despite Nurse Ron Attwood realising the situation had developed into one where it was regarded by some that I had done the damage; he raised Cain on the matter and arranged for a policeman from Crowthorne to come in and take a statement from me. It was Nurse Ron who enlightened me of the difficulties of storage in Broadmoor. There was no room. That was the reason for the social worker's procrastination at collecting my belongings; he had promised what he knew he could not deliver.

I was overjoyed when I heard Duggy Hunter was in trouble. There were then only a dozen people employed in admin, and one of them spotted that Mr Hunter had put in travelling expenses for visiting a patient's relatives on the same day that the relatives visited the patient in Broadmoor. Somebody acquired copy of a local newspaper account and it transpired that Mr Hunter, aged about forty five, had a lady friend in the same area as this patient and visited her frequently. He was fired. One patient was sorry to see the back of him. David Sims, in for murder and later moved from the parole ward for seeing Alan Reeve go over the wall and not reporting it, "Duggy would get my postal order each week for me to do the pools", he said sadly.

I did not have as many social workers as I did primary nurses – which could change six times in as many months – but, apart for one, they seemed to flit like unremembered shadows, bothering to make their reports and contributing nothing. One, Keith Lynn, went up in everybody's estimation by walking out of a meeting on the Block with the words, "I've had enough of this……..", and left to live in France with his dog. Paul, on the directive from the Chief Executive, went through the medical report of Dr Ropner who had interviewed me in Holloway Prison to commit me to Broadmoor and the gross errors acknowledged as such. One outstanding slur stated that I had worked for eight years only until I married. In fact I worked for twenty eight years and could prove it. I had thought that being able to discredit so many facts, the suppositions would be judged accordingly. Instead of marking the errors in the margin as is normal legal practice, the report was rewritten omitting the errors.

Until the Access to Medical Records Act was passed, I had had no sight of this document, I was never intended to see it and it took thirteen years for me to read what I was up against.

CHAPTER 4 - BROADMOOR

Christmas Routine and the New Year

Ten days before Christmas we are called to the day room and note strange staff on the ward wearing rubber gloves. The other day room is searched as we wait for the sniffer dogs with their handlers to go through our rooms. When the other day room is finished we move en masse into it and wait still more. One woman is called out mystified that, "The dog reacted in your room" and a more thorough search made of it, every item inspected and some innocuous talcum powder removed. This happened to me twice and I reached the conclusion that the dogs were tired and some show had to be made when nothing was found The dogs also reacted in front of the perfume cupboard in the corridor. Izzy's *Opium* perfume is blamed. Later we saw the dogs, a couple of spaniels, in the garden bounding across the flower beds. The search subdues us and there is a nasty feel.

It is Christmas Eve; after finishing touches to the ward decorations are made, the seven dwarfs look like models in a shop window. Such wasted talent. "The corridor windows weren't allowed to be opened last night for fear of spoiling them", Mitch says, "We roasted our end". Great excitement waiting to be judged, me dressed as Santa to welcome the judging committee and show them round. I hoped they wouldn't wander into the dining room, which is a bit sparse on the tinsel, all effort being made in the corridor and day rooms. Several of us have stuck our cards on the outside of our doors and walls and they add to the colour as the eye travels down the long corridor. Sister Sue has created a large turkey outside my door but the egg keeps dropping off and I am obliged to stick back the dropped feathers – pampas grass from the garden, picked in October in preparation for Xmas; Nurses Bob and John have been noble on a step-ladder, we are not allowed to do that in case we fall off; some staff say they're forbidden to stand on them too so we are in luck this year. A cardboard fireplace fronts the non-smoking dayroom alcove with a plate of mince pies for Santa that I keep my fingers crossed will survive the inspection. Nurse Anne-Marie runs in from Lancs to tell our staff "Your ward can't win". We do. And when Sister Sue comes on for the afternoon shift she is posturing and excited. It is obvious that our staff has won the competition with help from patients, rather than by the patients with help from staff.

One of the judges is the League of Friends Chairman, Julie Rule, and she enquires if we have received the music centre and I point to it. I refrain from stating what I think about it. Senior Nurse Webster looks on and grins – I've recently written to the Management pointing out the efforts they make to increase illness have sadly proved successful by flashing lights on us whilst we sleep and so on. Patient Julie runs up panting, "We've not got the video player yet". "We'll hire one for the holiday", says Webster. The holidays have already started, he'd better get a move on.

On Christmas Day the nurses in Seven Dwarfs outfit dispense tea and coffee to us in bed, the coffee being provided by us and the beaker placed outside our door the night previously. Our presents have been inspected for dangerous items and stored in brown

124

paper sacks with our names on and these are pushed into our rooms. Breakfast is called unusually early "for those who want it" and half the ward materialise at intervals in various stages of dress and undress. Traditionally we have fried eggs once a year but our staff who so lovingly take pains to decorate the ward and themselves in tinsel beards and wigs will not fry us eggs. They're not allowed to. We have mushrooms instead. Time was, when we ate en masse in the dining room, we had both.

The two wards can intermingle for a while and Alvada and I sit and chat over a coffee and goodies in the alcove outside her room. It's much quieter there. Every year one of the Embassy staff sends her a large box of the most gorgeous crystallised fruit and I am most appreciative of the gift to her. We're both saddened at Joan's absence; a year or two back there were five of us from another world; Joyce had once been a flare path guide in the WAAF and now lived in her own home, Margaret from Bath now lived with her sister; Joan; Alvada and I, we would annoy some by having little tea parties with tablecloth and fancy cakes. It was Joyce who organised such an event to celebrate the birth of my grandson; Joan always found something we others had forgotten, like a tablecloth and Wedgwood tea plates of which she had a supply. She sold me four tea plates for 25p the lot.

Joyce had once returned ashen-faced after a rare ward outing to the south coast. Alvada had been on the outward journey but her escape from the underwear counter at M & S had necessitated an earlier return for the rest than planned. An American who had been on her Embassy staff for many years,

Alvada had had the misfortune to contract fibroids and appendicitis. She was in Broadmoor for shooting the friend who introduced her to the surgeon who performed the urgent operation after his return from a South African holiday, three weeks after Alvada had been admitted to hospital. The surgeon was George Pinker, the Queen's gynaecologist. It was by accident, during a visit to her GP, Sir Ralph Southward, doctor to Prince Philip, that she read a letter from George Pinker stating that her healthy ovaries had been removed, "to prevent the spread of infection". If they were healthy, she reasoned, they could not spread infection but at the time there was a fashion for total hysterectomies. She wrote recorded delivery to all fifty-six members of the General Medical Council (GMC) demanding an enquiry and Pinker's expulsion from the medical register for his sadism. The result was a deputation from the GMC to the American Embassy demanding that Alvada be deported back to the States. If there could ever be more proof that she was a valuable employee, despite her age, there could be no higher accolade than the adamant refusal of her employers to obey the bidding of the Brits to get rid of her. She stayed with provisos. She would see the Embassy shrink who could not persuade her that her claims to being violated and mistreated were unfounded. At the age of fifty-two she had dreamed of having a child. Psychiatrists had relished this as a symptom of her insanity but the newspapers had glossed over this aspect to a large extent and intimated that the shooting was the result of a lesbian liaison. If it weren't so awful we could have enjoyed the differences between fact and fiction depicted in the British press when it related to us. She acquired the gun in S Africa after flying there for the day specifically for the purpose of its purchase claiming to need it in Zimbabwe. The gun was intended to shoot Pinker but instead she shot, at a bus stop in Knightsbridge, the friend who introduced her to him, "the traffic snarled up", Alvada said. The ugly, unrecognisable mug shot of her that appeared on TV, which could easily have enabled her to escape detection forever and a manic MP raving, "Murderers shouldn't be allowed on outings to the seaside" was indelible on my mind. I quite agree with him. The community should be protected from dangerous people but my idea of a danger to the public and the MP's was clearly rather different. I was not the only one who chided that she had shot the wrong person. She had lost her cool at a Knightsbridge bus stop when her friend told her yet again she should forget about her operation and stop being silly. This was one of the times of year she dreaded most, January and June with the New Year and Birthday Honours Lists. She always went through the newspapers meticulously for fear that old Pinks got a mention. "He'll get a knighthood," was her mantra. How she would have reacted if he had I do not know.

Her escape had been remarkable and her capture underlined yet again the variance of truth in press reports of such events. The media stated that she had been found in St Ermin's hotel trying the bedroom doors for a night's sleep. Joyce had been interested as her daughter had done some catering course there, "Trust Alvada to go somewhere classy", she had said.

"St Ermin's is in the same block as MI5", I said, remembering John Le Carre novels.

"What", said Alvada mystified when I told her, "I've never been there although I've heard of it. I caught a Green Line coach to Victoria, terrified I'd be picked up; I went to Westminster Cathedral for a while and listened to the choir practice and then stood by the exit from the banqueting hall at the Stars And Stripes Club. I stood in the alley, it wasn't pleasant. Some man tried to pick me up. Then I got in but the Manager found me and called the Police when he heard where I was from". The disgust on her face said it all. He didn't understand that she was trying to show the authorities that bumping off Pinker was not on her itinerary and she needed space to sleep for the night. She had escaped to prove she wasn't dangerous when free. It took a while for us to get the facts as on her return to the buildings she was sent to the Block and was out of circulation for a while. She did not know if the Stars & Stripes Club was the unofficial HQ of the CIA to match the St Ermin tale.

I was puzzled that an intelligent, astute, woman like Alvada who could accomplish both the *Telegraph* and *Times* crosswords in a morning, thought she could still be a mother at fifty something even though her then boy friend was a Police Superintendent, or Commissioner. She had shown me a report on her; among listed symptoms considered to be mental illness by the medical profession was that she had expected to have a child. She had told me that her grandmother had had a daughter when she was well into her fifties. "She was my grandfather's second wife, his first one died". The repetition of this fact, that her grandparents had had a child when beyond the normal age for such events, jogged my memory to something my maternal grandmother used to say and I had heard my mother recite: "When older parents have a child it's not theirs" and I told Alvada. She did not snap at me in protest that I didn't understand or her grandparents had defeated the maxim. She took the statement calmly, I could almost see her mind working as she realised that the woman she had always regarded as her aunt could well be her cousin. How sad that a woman who trusted and did not question what she was told by those in authority could make such an admirable civil servant but be led into such a difficult situation and land up in Broadmoor. The only other quote of my grandmother that I knew was, "Never tell a policeman you're going on holiday".

Alvada's ward had not made much effort to decorate, "Our staff have found their metier", I remarked, "but they look more like principal boys from *Peter Pan* than dwarfs".

I remember the Christmas my father was in hospital and my mother was looking after Aunty Joyce's City dwelling cat. My husband and I went to stay and were woken on Christmas morning with my mother in her boots and overcoat bearing us cups of coffee, wailing, "The cat's up the fir tree". It was a particularly scraggy fir tree, there was a splattering of snow on the ground, and the kitten's plaintiff meows wafted down to us as we gazed upwards. I rang the fire brigade to be told that they could not be called out for such an exigency without the authority of the man from the RSPCA. They gave me his phone number and his wife said that her husband was out tending a swan with a broken wing. He would call when he returned which he did; he duly arrived, took one look outside and said the cat's claws could not cope with the downward journey and he rang the fire brigade. My mother relaxed considerably at sight of the RSPCA man and said to John and me, "You go on. I'll phone when it's down and you can come back and collect me". . We were due at a drinks party with lunch afterwards with twenty others at the Fitz's before going to visit my father in hospital;   it was before the days of bans on drink driving.   We did as we were told but an hour and a half later there was no phone call from Mother to come and collect her so Uncle Leo bade me ring her.   "The fire engine's just leaving" she said in a happy voice. When I drew up she tottered out of the house to the car, "They've eaten all the mince pies and half the Christmas cake", she said happily, "and drunk nearly all the whiskey".   The cat was happy too but was not allowed out again.

One of the nicest Christmases I had in Broadmoor was shortly after I came when staff would play inmates at football on Boxing Day and those who wanted could go and watch.   Izzy, who was to become the biggest window smasher of them all when readmitted, had introduced me to David, who was thirteen years younger than me (Izzy later died of Crohn's disease and was buried within the walls).   "I'm old enough to be your mother", I had said when he asked if we could sit together at a social, "I'm a hairy baby", he replied. He said he was going to watch the match and would I like to walk round with him.   The men were allowed to take thermos flasks to the Sports Field and David's was filled with beer.   This had been brought in plain cans, the labels removed – it could never have happened on the female wing – and represented a sympathetic staff man along the line.   I provided home made mince pies and pastries brought in by a friend whose mother had made them specially.   I felt at peace walking round the perimeter munching and swigging at intervals in the frosty air.   We were breaking the rules, or rather David was and whoever brought the beer in, but it was harmless.   Boxing Day football matches have not happened for a long time, only the most skeleton of staff are available over holiday periods and there are not enough to play a game, let alone be spared to act as escorts for events. Today there is segregation of the sexes and no food, not even food parcels from Harrods are allowed in.

There's a card from David now transferred to Ashworth away from his few relations in the south of England. I knew he could not expect many visits so, as a way of assuaging Spiritualist Bill for the ban on his visiting me I asked David if he would like Bill to visit him. Bill was agreeable; "I can just hop on the bus from here", he wrote me. The visit not only proved fruitful, David had his first day out in thirty five years thanks to Bill having him home to tea and they enjoyed walking along the beach at West Kirby. Their friendship lasted till Bill died – he would say "passed away to the other side".

As soon as the festivities are over and the decorations taken down, the tension sets in again. Tracy B cut herself badly and is on the Block, she's a perky little sparrow with cropped hair but for a lock of perhaps six hairs at the back of her head. Wonderful artist. The gang took to watching videos in fast succession making it impossible for Eug to watch *Home And Away*. She was furious. She took a chair to her room and used it as a weapon to smash up as much of it as possible. As she bashed the staff came running. Ma and I remembered a previous occasion when Eug. was on the ward downstairs and told everyone in the dining room to "Get out" before picking up the television and flinging it at the windows. Crash. After such an outburst it was amazing how quickly she calmed down; she was led away looking most docile, the humble look descending at great speed after such a display of passion.

Next day a friend phoned to say she was visiting but the weather is so awful that I had given up and was contemplating taking a bath when she arrived. It had taken her ten minutes to locate the main entrance.

At school the tutor tells us that three Broadmoor nurses on the reserve list have been called up as medics for the Gulf War. We are intrigued. Is this to be a psychological war? Will the injured be informed that their wounds are solely in the mind. Deadline is midnight tomorrow.

There's an altercation in the sewing room where it's Georgie's turn to make the tea; Shiela ever provocative says it tastes like pee. Nellie also complains and receives a cup poured over her. It is Nellie who goes back to the ward to change her clothes. "Georgie's off it", says Shiela who insists, "she's been crouching over the radio", inferring that she is supposed to have received messages from it. I retired to the quiet of the loo and missed Marge tipping a cup of cold water over Georgie who thumps Tracy. Alarm bell pressed. Staff pour in.

In my post there is some literature from the Schizrenia Association who maintain that all human behaviour can be cured with a pill, the snag being that the discovery of such a pill has still to be made and rests with donations from readers. The organisation complains that relatives go to great pains to have their loved ones committed then the psychiatrists let them out before they are cured. I remember hearing a User Group, from the early days of the psychiatric protest movement, deplore that MIND meetings always had parents complaining their loved ones weren't committed fast enough. Some

132

things come in different packaging but don't change very much. There is also some literature from WISH (Women In Special Hospitals), which I pass on to Mitch, and Ma who beam happily. Gay or lesbian literature is more their scene than mine.

We are not allowed to stay up to see in the New Year but a piper comes round, his Auld Lang Syne echoing in the night breeze. When we have the keys to our doors we are allowed to stay up and see the old year out and the new in and watch the fireworks at Sandhurst through the day room windows.

It is Wednesday , 16 January 1991 and we are at war with Iraq. At school the Vicar's wife shows us a film on anti-Semitism and asks us to indicate where we would like a discussion. Bushy-haired George has the video stopped in the middle. What does George wish to discuss. Ponderously he says, "Why do Jews talk through their nose a lot?" which clearly disconcerted the tutor. She rallied with, "Well people do have traits, or characteristics and they do have large noses" to which George said, "Is their language really Gibberish".

"Yiddish", I said and George receded back into silence.

Visits are now back on and in the Central Hall. The waiter at our table today is Mark; he came up to us with two mega-cones rejected by someone to our right. We ate them. A meal in themselves. Tepid drinks again. My friend disconcerted me by saying she would visit me more often; for some reason this saddened me as this meant that she did not think I would get out and she was cheering me up. She blanched when I told her that I had written to a TV chat show host whose subject that day had been prison suicides. One of the TV speakers had insisted that prisoners were issued with razor blades to cut themselves and a PO man had replied that prisoners usually hung themselves. Clearly this is a non-u topic but I was struck, particularly as the situation worsened considerably, by the fact that although the Second World War had claimed the lives of forty- two million people, and injured countless more, I had not known any of them. Already I had lost count of the number of deaths that had occurred in Broadmoor since my arrival.

That evening I phoned my daughter to hear she was waiting for a date and finance for her op; their local hospital were on alert for the Gulf War, a ward there being closed last year for lack of nurses. I should be out of here looking after her.

Terry is missing; rumour says she has gone to hospital with stomach ache but Dee says she was told not to say anything but Terry had a fall and was knocked unconscious. Marge says it was in the bathroom. Yesterday Dr Ghosh had seen her to say Friern Barnet would accept her within a week and this has given her the courage to speak out and break the silence and as many rules as she can manage. She takes her Walkman's to work and meals and is a big bore with the squeaks from her earphones. Maggy S, previously determined to get married in Broadmoor to another patient says she will now wait till she gets out. There have been a spate of weddings; whereas those normally conducted outside receive acclaim, there are misgivings about those couples in Broadmoor who marry. The press relished the news and always printed lurid accounts of the crimes which had led to the convictions so that one couple went to undue lengths, each changing their names several times beforehand. Thus if the press knew about the marriage, the informant could be pinned down and sued. It was acknowledged that life outside could be lonely, with the facts of a Broadmoor stay concealed to avoid embarrassment, so relations between male and female patients were poignant, each seeking security. It was also realised that few women could contract a respectable marriage outside Broadmoor and several men who had been convicted of rape would figure more respectably and stand a better chance of release if they could show to have a wife. Marriages could not be consummated within the walls so a wedding was a non-event in the context of the real meaning.

At roll call, now advanced to 8.30 p.m. Marge remarks of a woman on TV, "She looks like Mrs B in the sewing room".
"Come off it Marge, that one's a Madam". Marge laughs. "Well Mrs B does call us her girls doesn't she". The size of our rooms can be compared to those for the concubines in Istanbul's harem and the female wing at Broadmoor is situated on the eastern perimeter but there the comparison ceases.

I'm concerned at an interview Dr Chandra Ghosh had with me. She asked me for details of my medication – surely the files gave this information. "And Joan", she said emphatically, "When we cleared up her things there was a letter stating that her husband had died". She stared at me but I made no comment and the meeting ended. I assume she had heard me say that if Joan had been allowed to leave as she wished to live with her friend she would still be alive. The interview preyed on my mind. There was a routine whereby OT staff were advised of any problem experienced by a patient so that they could help if the need arose when the inmate was at "work"; they also read through the ward reports when they collected patients for the work areas. If the death of Joan's husband's had been known to Broadmoor note would have been made of it in the file and daily report. When I next saw staff from the Sewing Room I told them the story and asked if they knew anything. They were surprised. "No. We didn't know Joan's husband had died", they choroused, they would have remembered something like that. I even mentioned it to her ward sister doing an extra shift on ours, she would have known if anything unusual had been discovered in Joan's belongings. "No," she said clearly amazed, " and I don't recall anything like that being in the report. I don't think there was mention of it at the inquest either". It was all very odd particularly as incoming mail is censored, (for some years outgoing letters were not examined but incoming has always been opened), one of the stated reasons for doing so was in case of death an inmate might be upset and require comfort in the form of the Chaplain. On one occasion I was called to the office to be handed a letter by Sister Jane who soulfully told me, "I am afraid I have bad news. Stanley has died". I was mystified. The letter she handed me disclosed that the father of a friend had died and another acquaintance had written to advise me. "He was an Income Tax Inspector" I told her. On several occasions where relatives had died, letters were delivered to me without comment. If Joan had received such a letter there should have been some note about it although, admittedly, it did not always happen.

The year before Chandra Ghosh took over the female wing the movement rate for one hundred and twenty women had been six.   Dr Ghosh moved twenty-two in her first year although several came back to Broadmoor unhappy where they had been sent and even more unhappy to have to start once more at the bottom of the system when they came back. The staff were alarmed at the work involved with a faster turnover and disturbance this caused and this formed one of the bases for their dislike of her. She intensely disliked her staff; I had difficulty believing the extent of this antipathy that was told to me by the friend who visited me and gave the doctor a lift afterwards.   We were aware that our new psychiatrist preferred to interview patients alone; staff preferred that one of them was present at the interview thereby inhibiting the patient's full disclosure of ward occurrences. To be away from the ward staff Dr Ghosh tried to arrange to see patients in the Sewing Room where there was hardly space for us to sit, let alone conduct an interview.   Sewing Room staff did not like her for taking no interest in their work and yet trying to use their area to see her patients.   Most patients regarded the new arrival as a distinct improvement on the previous Australian, described on more than one occasion as a lounge lizard and who, we are told, has now died and felt there was now some hope of release.   For ever I will remember a diminutive figure wearing full length fur coat stepping across the potholes in the forecourt, her sari making ripples across the puddles. She did not get her feet wet or splash her sari. I never met another professed communist who wore such a variety of leather and fur coats.

In the morning the nurse forgets which ward she's on and slings the lock when she wakes us so the door can't shut and bangs with the wind. "Oh", says the nurse, "I've lost my head this morning" and un-slings it. At one time it was considered a safety precaution to have all the locks slung so all the doors banged but I could never see the sense in it; after some years the routine was discontinued when greater leniency overcame the greater unreasonable harshness. I settle back to sleep. Am just thinking that I should get up when there's a shuffling in the corridor, a knock on my door. It's Jane, her knees have given her trouble for some time and she uses the door frame for support. "We're at war", she says.

"Who fired the first shot?" I say.

"We did. At five o'clock this morning our planes bombed chemical installations in Iraq".

Sister Irene asks me: "Which side are you on?". I was startled but realised she was not referring to the Gulf. "I don't have a side", I say when I understand she was referring to the recent argument about closing the kitchen and wash room doors at medicine times. A Senior Nursing Officer has decreed they and the one to the ward downstairs remain open. We had not been told of specifics but understand there is a difference of opinion amongst staff, some of whom are concerned that they will lose authority, power. It was a conflict that was to mar our increased freedom and lasted for the next fifteen years.

"There were seventeen of them wandering around" Sister says with a shudder and I realise "them" means us patients and seventeen of us had decided not to eat in the dining room. Thus they were sitting listening to music, watching TV or fast asleep. Seventeen. It had been decided that meals should not

138

be compulsory – there were weight problems which had to be addressed and it was agony for some to have to sit and watch others eat when they should not – so that if some opted to eat and others did not staff were then required to monitor the whole ward, not just the dining area. I see Sister is frightened of losing a grip on us. She is happy only with everybody sitting confined to the day room where she can see them. I feel people are less trouble if allowed to go to sleep in their rooms. I was amazed and saddened that she did not want the doors between the wards remaining open during meal times and she was fighting to find some way to stop it happening.

For all the time until the 1970's the doors had been open between the wards;   the girls would get up and go to the ward downstairs for a chat, smoke and drink before getting dressed to go out to breakfast in the dining room, then in a nearby building.   Without warning or incident security was tightened. Some staff and several patients had been in tears when a steel gate had been erected at the top of the stairs to restrict ward movement, staff could not imagine how they could contain the ward with so little freedom and inevitably restrictions became stricter and stricter. The point had been reached where for some years the residents had not even been allowed a light for a cigarette before they were dressed on their own ward, let alone wandering off in a dressing gown to another. Now it was proposed that the ward door be open permanently which was producing more tears by staff in opposition to the proposal.

At school a patient shouts, "Why shouldn't Saddam Hussein have a coastline, other countries have.   And he's only a little country to be bombed like that".   As in so many matters there is a difference of opinion about who should have what.

New Year's Eve sees pay awards for the public sector. A Grade A Nurse pay increases by £755; consultant by £5,600, teacher £1500, top Civil Servants by £10,000 and judges by 9.5 – 12.1% several having a hundred K to start with. I feel very poor. Perhaps this will bring an end to our broken nights, cancelled visits, arguments about open doors and slow movement rate to block the system. In all my working experience I only once asked for a pay increase and I was so disgusted that I had to do it I left when I got it. Surely some better method of awarding the public sector could be found than the apparent necessity to disrupt and therefore blackmail public services.

I do not cheer up even though Alvada is delighted her gynaecologist receives no mention in the New Year honours. I've just heard Cathy slipped two weeks back and broke three teeth and her jaw. She was kept on the ward a couple of days before being sent out to hospital. She's now like another girl on the ward whose jaw keeps growing unnaturally so her teeth don't meet; both have their jaws wired up. I feel happier when my son-in-law phones to leave a message that my Daughter's op went well and nothing awful was discovered. He's taking time off to look after the children. I should be doing it. We throw snowballs in the corridor.

The Hereford probation officer cancels his visit as the roads are so bad and more snow promised. The Sewing Room was late calling, the reason being that the OT head had given them a pep talk. According to one of them they were to talk more among themselves. We are all puzzled. An OT tutor is sitting in to watch one of them who is taking a qualification to increase her pay. The nurse is required to show Georgie how to make a stuffed toy. "Patient showing staff", murmurs the tutor with a smile but we don't laugh. I am told that I have turned down the opportunity to work in the garden and that I wanted to be alone; interpreted this is jargon for no work place can be found for me other than the sewing room which is not suitable as the noise of the sewing machines and radio worsens my tinnitus. My suggestion that I work in the library was ignored.

Lord Lane releases a couple accused and found guilty of torturing to death their young son on grounds that there was no evidence to show which one did it! Another instance of the guilty going free (after two years). Not for the first time I wonder if I should feel proud that I am being detained so long. The Judicial system releases the guilty. The innocent have their own reward, it is said.

Nurse Bob calls me to the office to ask when I last saw my suitcase, now found to be missing when I wanted to lend it to a patient going into an outside hospital for a few days.. "Eighteen months back" I said.

A hairdresser is now missing from the salon – she is now a nurse. We all pale at the prospect, she is a very good hairdresser but we doubt her capabilities as a care assistant. She will be one of those who asks, "Can they have this? Can they do that?" She needs the extra money to buy a house. This change of occupation after being sent on a £500 course to learn how to do men's hair, "No she didn't. The staff blocked it", said the other hairdresser, "it never happened". I gather the men have to rely on each other or a member of staff for barbering. For reasons of security the ward scissors on the female wing are too blunt for hair cutting although few of us mind this difference of self-sufficiency in the sexes.

Current Affairs at school was visited by a group of prison officers from Lewes Prison and today a student psychologist called David sat in and also attended the typing class. What does he hope to gain from this "observation"? In addition to these and regular visitors we had a flux of VIP's. Andrew McKay MP for Bracknell came in to the classroom escorted by Alan Franey, Chief Executive and Les Martin the Head Tutor. We asked mundane questions like how soon will the oil fires started by the Iraqis in Kuwait be contained and how friendly was the local green policy. I mentioned the time I had sat in the visitors' gallery along with foreign tourists to be embarrassed at the few MP's on view and the ones there were had their feet up. I had tried to explain to those around- mostly visitors from abroad - that most of the work was done back-stage in committee. Was I correct? Alan Franey dived into the corridor to suppress his mirth, everyone laughed.

CHAPTER 5 - BROADMOOR

The Royal Visit – 7 March 1991

We have difficulty believing it. Princess Di is coming to Broadmoor and visiting the ward downstairs. Alvada refuses to take part in the proceedings and meet her. Doreen agrees to give her Royal Highness tea. There's nothing like a Royal visit to smarten things up, the cleaners are on the ward in droves. Joan maintained that patients' rooms had not been decorated for over twenty years so I trust the one Doreen is presenting refreshments in is passable. The noisy leaf/pigeon dropping picker has been and gone from the courtyard, there isn't a scrap of paper that dares to be seen flying in the wind; some of us gather in the dining room to watch the bustle and I shout through the window to young Dr Murphy as he lopes towards the building. "You can't walk on it. It's been cleaned. You've got to fly over it". We see a movement on the horizon, which produces more yelling, "They're coming", and watch the Chief Executive Alan Franey and entourage escort the Princess wearing a green suit to our building where she meets the patients. I was surprised there was no lady in waiting. Lady Diana is a very uncluttered princess. She is reputed to have remarked that the smell of wet paint was a usual herald for a Royal visit but in Broadmoor she was assailed by the smell of fresh tarmac, which explained the activity to cover up the worst potholes and the arrival of a path that previously had been muddied grass. Later we watch the news and see her greeted by schoolchildren outside waving Union Jacks.

On a later occasion she visited the new education centre and I greeted her in the computer room. A male patient was very bold and told her, "You married the wrong man". She was very lovely.

My Hereford friend came in the morning with news that Dr Chandra Ghosh is having injunctions on her over Anne P and Dr Pamela Taylor at SHSA is blocking the release of me and others. When I relay this to Mitch she screams that I'm stirring it and she hopes I choke on my fish and chips. I speak to Sister Sue who advises, "Write to Pamela Taylor and tell her and ask where this leaves you". She added, "I wouldn't know who had the largest wooden spoon". Ghosh had described Taylor as "vile".

A symptom of psychopathic disorder, called playing politics by some, is a tendency to manipulates others and it is patent that many psychiatrists do have their patients' characteristics, like dogs resembling their owners. I was being manipulated, pulled in several directions by different factions but it did not do to dwell on the subject, bitterness is not a happy companion.

Ma is in a talkative mood. "I'm in Broadmoor because of Dr Loucus" she says with a grin. "I was really grateful to him for getting me here". She would otherwise have been in a male prison; the fact that she was on the female wing in a Special Hospital showed once again the flexibility of the Mental Health Act when it suits. It is normal for Broadmoor psychiatrists to interview those destined for Broadmoor and one ward sister had been under the impression that Dr Lecouteur had interviewed everybody on the ward prior to admittance. I had done a check to discover that one only out of thirty-eight had in fact been seen by him prior to arrival. At least Ma had been seen by a psychiatrist from Broadmoor even if he was responsible for sex offenders on the male side and he had been the subject of a TV documentary on the subject of his hormone implants. Two patients had sued him for growing breasts, which had to be removed surgically leaving them with no nipples. By my reckoning Dr Loucus' treatment of sexual deviants made the doctor a sex offender.

Princess Diana's visit has been described in the press as "Princess of Wales visits Broadmoor and shakes hand with a killer" – Tommy Knight, later to commit suicide in an outside hospital, his girlfriend did the same in here. He maintained, "I should think it did Broadmoor some good that publicity; must have been a press handout, couldn't have been the Palace". He's several packets of fags better off as staff have asked him to draw pictures of their children. Bad publicity is still publicity.

I don't know who was responsible for it, I suspect the school tutor for whom I had typed his father's biography, but Nurse Bob called me to the office and told me I had been offered a job in the school office. It was a breakthrough. I was the first woman in Broadmoor to be given what is reckoned to be "a decent job". The men always had the jobs in the library, shop, and all the occupations that in prison would be called Trusties' duties. On the female wing it was usual for ward work to be given to smokers as they created the most uproar when they ran short of money. The competition to secure means to earn some extra pennies was frequently low and anybody with a job that somebody else wanted could have a rough time. I doubted there was anyone else on the ward with the ambition for this job with a little office with me alone that earned £25 per month. No more noisy sewing room exacerbating my tinnitus or heavy lifting on the ward. There was a snag in that I am not in the least technically-minded but luckily there was Mike Ananin the IT tutor who smilingly advised me and Terry, a computer whiz kid, who was on hand; his skill earned 50p to my 43ph and he was patience personified when teaching me how to use the computer and dot matrix printer with the programme he had devised for the time-tables. In a normal school timetables are set for the year and remain unchanged for that time. Broadmoor Education Centre is somewhat different.

Socials, education, work areas and church, in addition to their recognised function also served as venues for boy meets girl. It was difficult, if they were concerned on the matter, for the teachers and staff to determine the actual reason for application to join a certain class, but the start and finishing of liaisons could be reflected in the school timetable. The other reasons for changes included the desperation of an inmate for an opportunity to escape work area and the ward so would join up for a class for which they quickly tired particularly if their attention span was low, institution of short-course lectures of, say, six weeks, change of ward, being a new admittance, leaving, and I stumbled across a further need to make changes. "Terry", I said after a few weeks, "there are an awful lot of name changes. Mitch is now Ricky something and there's a flood of Mohammeds from Jo Bloggs and the women are getting married". Terry obligingly amended the menu to accommodate this latest craze so I could type in the original name, the new one with the name of house and ward and the entire set of sheets be altered automatically. I draw a veil over the occasion I left the printer unattended and the reams of paper that became entangled with the machine……. Plus I had great difficulty being able to fit the memo sheets to match the spaces provided. How Terry and his pals could fiddle about arranging the type one and a half centimetres from the top of the page on the screen and twenty point three millimetres from the left and so much from the right margin I cannot imagine. I solved that one by ignoring the stack of printed memo pads supplied by the Print Shop and created my own. I typed in "To;" and "From:" on clean sheets.

Prior to the advent of computers great effort had been taken to prevent too many changes to the timetables, the female wing particularly was renowned for being hard line because those in authority could not cope. Before the arrival of computers I had helped the previous Head Tutor who set up the Education Centre, Ieuan Williams, manually type up a timetable and it was a fiddly exercise. I could see that it was expedient to keep the sheets static but a result of the policy of making a patient stay in a class they didn't want was two-fold; arguments between reluctant pupil and escort staff, "I told Dr Le Couteur I didn't want to go to maths six months ago. I hate it" and a larger class list than met reality so other figures did not tally. Now the changes were marked off by staff on a master copy and on Fridays I would make the amendments – frequently over 100 of them – and send copies to each ward, Radio Control, escort staff, the Allocations Officer, and then pin a master copy on the school notice board and another in Les Martin's, Head Tutor's room. How much of it was necessary I could only conjecture. It was Mike who fixed the computer when it would not print capitals, "It does that sometimes" he said reassuringly – probably thinking "Oh dear". I was also required to keep track of the books in the school's library and order the stationery

In the summer the escort, particularly Nurse Shirley, would keep taking the room temperature with the view to announcing the closure of the school. She would hover anxiously – eagerly – waiting for the gauge to rise the last degree. The Education Centre was expecting to move to one newly built, on the site of the vacated doctors' quarters opposite Kent House with lovely views. The doctors were being relocated to what was called Fantasy Island, the new admin block where their activities, if sitting and chatting to each other could be so termed, could not be observed and commented on by male patients in the overlooking houses nearby. Les was emphatic that the new quarters would have a sloping roof and air conditioning. No more hoping the temperature gauge would rise so we could all go home. The new venue would be quieter, the noise from lorries arriving and backing from delivering goods to the canteen was a distraction particularly during examinations. The present building would be used by Estates and then converted to house medical records.

The Education Centre had been started when a fourteen year old was sent to Broadmoor. It had now grown to include four resident tutors who linked with the wards to such an extent a third of their time was taken with meetings, not teaching, and several part-timers. They were all very nice and pleasant. The one fly was Bert. To start with he was dubious that a female could work in his school – he was the security man in charge of the escorts. He would send Nurse

Shirley down to glower if a male inmate dared to talk to me at the door but he gradually thawed and ultimately put in a hook for me to hang my coat up. His daughter was sweet. She worked as a domestic on our ward and I was amazed they were related. It was always wise to be careful in conversation with staff as so many nice ones were connected to the most unlikely people.

The education unit had grown to be an integral, essential, part of Broadmoor's routine and I realised that what I had missed most since my arrival was an academic atmosphere. 'O' level examinations, to become GCSE's were catered for, 'A' levels covered by correspondence courses, for OU courses, part-funded by the individual, the rest by Broadmoor, a special tutor visited. Then there was the Koestler.

Arthur Koestler gave his name to an award scheme which was started by his friends prompted by boredom in jails, of which Koestler had experienced three, one in Spain under sentence of death by garrotting whilst a newspaper correspondent, the second in France for passport offences and the third in Pentonville for the same reason. Pentonville was the worst. The Home Office approved the scheme so once a year prisoners submitted works of art, literature and so on and an exhibition of the best items arranged. Although it is not a prison residents of Broadmoor were allowed to submit entries. To start with, the Activity Centre (later to become the Social & Recreation Department) would handle the entries, which were comparatively few in comparison with the number of people detained. Les Martin at the school was keen to take on the organising and from his encouragement the number and quality of entries from Broadmoor increased dramatically. From just a trickle I had to keep an annual list of over a hundred entries and notify the growing numbers of winners. I would type up the hand-written poetry and prose for those unable to type their own to present it as best I could. Nurse Shirley was disgusted at one piece. "You shouldn't have to type that", she exclaimed. "It's art", I said.

We all got a kick out of it and Les would arrange for the transport department to take the items – some from the carpentry shop were really good but enormous – to whichever prison was receiving them. His office would be crammed with boxes. The increased prison population was reflected by The Koestler Award Scheme, which grew to a very professional size, the venue for its exhibition growing too. Those items that were not sold by permission of the creators were returned and this included all the writing. I kept my returned files on top of my wardrobe in a large highly coloured box that had contained M & S flowers sent in by my daughter. It became so heavy I could hardly lift it. The day came when rules were introduced that prohibited the keeping of anything on the top of cupboards or on the floor. Paperwork allowance was limited to one file, clothes to a maximum of forty items, fifteen on some wards, the surplus was either sent out to be stored or destroyed. But it hadn't yet happened. These were the halcyon days of 1991 before we learned that in each of our files was a letter from Broadmoor's solicitors, Reid Minty, advising RMO's that, in the event of inquest brought about by forced medication the RMO would be exonerated as forced drugging was allowed under the Mental Health Act.

CHAPTER 6 - BROADMOOR

Pastimes

When I first arrived in Broadmoor the game of bowls played a significant part of summer activity, socials and indoor games being discontinued from April till the end of September. The then female wing-nursing officer was Miss Dean, a keen county bowls player, who encouraged the game and probably if she had retired before I arrived I would never have played. The second terrace of York House garden had a four-rink bowling green and for matches when outside teams visited there was a supply of grey skirts and white blouses made in the Sewing Room for the home team to wear. It was not long before I was introduced to the game and told I was playing in a match. The staff picked the female teams. There was a scramble for the cupboard which housed the equipment and I landed with a skirt several sizes too large, a very uncomfortable pair of flat shoes with soles that did not mark the precious green, cut and watered specially, and a set of woods that must have been circa 1930 and too large for my hands. It was a most enjoyable afternoon with tea and the visitors were kind in coaching us beginners on the techniques of the game. I overheard a nurse whisper to a group of the visiting ladies, "I'll show you to the loo and tell you what they're in for", and there was a nod in the direction of a very good bowls player in for infanticide.

There was an internal championship and the finalists played before an audience of the entire of York House with dignitaries like the psychiatrist and certain selected male patients, followed by presentation of bouquets of flowers to the participants and a barbecue or social in the dining room. It was a really pleasant civilised afternoon, one difficult to equate with the reputation of Broadmoor. I was in the finals twice and jokingly said that "J Cresswell" on the cup was my husband's name. The male side had two three-rink greens on the terrace and on Saturdays there would be mixed matches and tea in the Central Hall. The men picked their own teams and selection of females, which, like selection for their football team, depended as much on friendship with the selector than ability to play. Female bowls came to a sudden, fast, end with the retirement of Miss Dean. I was surprised at the ill feeling by some staff at the game. "Having to watch that for hours on end" and so on. The height of rebellion came with the bravery of a few of them dancing across the green. Not even the enthusiasm of two sisters who were both good club standard could revive the game, the weight of hostility by staff who could not be bothered to get the key to unlock the cupboard to get the bowls out saw to that. "It's a security risk", one said, "We have some very sick patients here.

The collapse of my back when I found I could not bowl a wood to the end of the green finished my attending the mixed matches for some years, and female participation petered out but I did play some evenings on the sports field with David who was my dancing partner for some while. He had quite a reputation, the roof several times, a court appearance whilst at Broadmoor, involvement with a girl on the female wing who sat on his knee after making a hole in the crutch of her tights, and a father, a Lloyd's Underwriter, who had visited to say, "Well son, you wont walk in dog shit here". On paper he appeared terrible but he was intelligent, good looking, and in many ways we shared the same views. Sports Field was Tuesdays and Thursdays in the summer, provided it didn't rain and staff were available and willing to escort us. Sometimes we would get there to be told that there weren't enough staff to monitor the bowling green – a recently constructed £32K affair without means of watering and built on the wrong foundations. But the exercise and open air was refreshing and it was a pleasant break.

Tennis was played for a while but making the sports field female only , rather than having tennis for females and allowing the men to watch and chat with their girl friends, meant that only a few girls wanted to play.   Security then decreed that no less than six people be escorted to the sports field. "It takes four to play tennis", I protested but common sense at Broadmoor is in short supply and it was only the stoicism of Sister Brookes (she who had been laid on to inspect the Block and see the girls were fed when they had been left without for days on end) that got me any tennis at all.   When she was on duty, four of us played; when she was not, we hardly went at all.   She was sympathetic to those with medical problems as her mouth was wry and sagging from an operation on her ear. After Nan left she and I would frequently stroll round the garden together; it was she who told me how grateful the staff were for my collaring a *News of the World* reporter when he came round and telling him that the central heating system had not worked in a third of York House for fifteen years.   I had pointed to the £20 a sq. yard carpet and told him not to be taken in by that.   The other end of the corridor was freezing.   Shortly afterwards efforts were made to rectify the problem. The west end of the corridor was always cooler than the hothouse end and I always opted where possible to have a room there. It was certainly a big improvement on the arctic conditions existing prior to the heating being fixed.

There had been no hint in the reporter's article that he had listened to anything I said. A double-page spread pictured the very nice room on the parole ward of Eleanor Buckingham who had refused the offer of a housekeeper's job to a village priest and preferred to stay at Broadmoor. She was visibly shaken how her crime of murdering her child thirty years previously was splashed across the paper; I wondered how short public memories were and if anyone would recognise her in the street. She ultimately died in Broadmoor and was buried there.

There was also swimming. Broadmoor provided swimming costumes for those without and I quickly became grateful that, considering how many of my belongings had been pilfered or gone missing, three swim suits survived. I gave two away, the third lasted me for the next twenty-five years. Twice a week, in the summer evenings, whatever the weather, swimming was available in the small pool donated by the League of Friends. The then Medical Superintendent, Dr Patrick McGrath had described it as "a hip bath" but it accommodated all the women that wanted to go. The disadvantage for the women was not the size of the pool but its situation at the bottom of Essex (to be renamed Berkshire) House, the men's parole block. The men blatantly stood on their terrace, some with binoculars, watching us. One, David Simms, had a ringside view of us. He would loll on the wall by the pool wearing his swimming trunks with his potbelly overflowing. He was the swimming pool attendant responsible for its cleanliness and, perhaps I misheard, he was our lifeguard. It was he who collared me, a new female patient, to say, "You want to get yourself a boyfriend then you can come to our parole dances in the winter." He was Nan's friend and had one of the beautifully tended allotments on the terrace between Essex House (to be renamed Berkshire House) and the pool. He would send over samples of the apricots he had grown and packets of Maybeline eyeliner, which Nan adored. If allowed she would go to bed wearing her thick make-up which saved re-applying it in the morning.

The dressing up for parole dances was amazing. As the girls lined up to be escorted to the event there would be a higher proportion of long evening dresses than at the Savoy and this lasted for many years until ballroom dancing became a thing of the past and disco dancing took over completely. In the winter there were socials and games evenings, one that comprised table tennis and the other cards and board games. Like most mixed functions these were mainly opportunities for cuddles, which the staff endeavoured to curtail but it was obvious that few women played either table tennis or board games. They wanted music that interfered with those involved in serious games of chess or bridge and these get-togethers were later abandoned.

The office I occupied in the new Education Centre looked onto the bowling green and I felt wistful seeing the men playing there on Wednesday afternoons. After a while I asked Martin Youett, the patient who organised it, if there was chance of a game and he looked at me hard and said, "If the men don't mind" and so I played on his rink. For several years I was the only woman and the difficulty I had during the first season getting to the match was enormous. Although I worked in the Education Centre by the side of the bowling green I was not allowed on Wednesday afternoons to go there first for an hour before the match started at 3 p.m. I could not cross the five yards as the ticket Bert had didn't allow this. I had to go straight from the ward. The ward had to provide an escort. There was one nurse, who later retired to Portugal, who loved fresh air and a reason to escape the over-heated ward, and she would engineer every opportunity to take me over and partake of tea in the Central Hall – usually chicken and chips or similar. The trouble was that she was not always on duty so sometimes I did not turn up at all, other times I was late. The second year different arrangements were made and staff from Soc. & Rec. would collect; they equipped me with a white jacket marked "Patmoor Bowling", a proper grey skirt purchased from a sports shop, a new white blouse and the woods were of modern manufacture. The teams were always smartly turned out, the men wore grey flannels and white shirts.

After a while I struck up a partnership with Peter Crozier who had also been placed under a Section 43 whilst in prison prior to being sent to Broadmoor, his explanation being an accepting, "It's the Mental Health Act" which did not satisfy me as others had been sent to the same destination without this unpleasantness. Peter and I won the handicap pairs for bowls on a couple of occasions; after his discharge resulting from two stressful tribunals each lasting a week or more with statements of four hundred pages, he played in his County's second team until he died. By this time the finals were no longer a grand occasion with chairs round the green and the Medical Superintendent present.   Neither the renamed Medical Director nor Chief Executive found time for such occasions. Finals were very low-key events with only the Soc & Rec. staff but enjoyable all the same.

For a while other women played in bowls matches but their behaviour of having cuddles on the green with their loved ones did not go down well with visitors or staff. The words, "You'll be on camera" were frequent and several of us conjectured if there were private showings of juicier cuddles like in the pornography section of the British Museum which sported private parties of MP's, judges and so on. There would be a bowls and cricket dinner and dance to mark the end of the season when trophies would be presented but the number of matches fell from a regular two a week to an occasional trickle of the patriotic after the Management banned visitors from smoking – the home team could smoke, visitors could not – and increased security which made visiting onerous.

The Broadmoor magazine, *The Chronicle* had been started in 1944 at a time when there was severe paper shortage in the land. At school we were required to write on the top and underneath the bottom line as well as on the covers of our exercise books and every scrap of paper was saved for recycling. It seems very typical that Broadmoor, like water shortages in times of national drought, should flout the trend and choose that time to start a magazine.   Over the years it fluctuated in tone thereby reflecting the spirit of the many editors and the politics in power.   It is a strange facet of the Conservative Party that there seems to be a greater freedom of expression when it is in government and that this can be reflected in an obscure penal magazine.   When I arrived the articles struck me as ingratiating, thick with thanks to staff for allowing a function and so on and full of news from the football field. I did my best to break from this servile role model and my first piece was a story about a dog called Boyce (the name of the female wing psychiatrist) who had broken loose to knock my mother's clothes prop over and dirty the washing. A true story but I never knew the Great Dane's real name. When the magazine office moved to the Education Centre it became far more regular and the Print Shop did its utmost to publish monthly on time; my bowls partner, Peter Crozier, although never an editor, contributed many brilliant articles with a legal and satirical slant. The magazine came to a staggering halt with the introduction of the Tilt Report and the Blair/Labour government when few could face the newly introduced restrictions going with the job of editor. From thereon no inmate was allowed to print their own computer work and all copies had first to be sent to the appropriate ward manager for vetting; there were frequent occurrences of the addressee being away and the work taking some weeks to be handed on.

After Tilt all mixed functions were stopped, work areas and Education traumatised; the Sports Field, expensively equipped with cameras, abandoned as too far to go in the event of an emergency, and segregation was such that even though a mixed bowling team would come in I was not allowed to play. I consoled myself that I had won the men's single final the year before the ban was imposed. Somehow what happened to the game of bowls at Broadmoor symbolised the regime as a whole. Great enthusiasm, expense, hands-on interest by the Management, a hard-line interpreted ruling followed by disinterest and decline.

CHAPTER 7 - BROADMOOR

Change of Direction

I had a visit yesterday so missed meeting the new writing tutor who was coming in for a few weeks. My friend visited the next day too and told me she'd given Dr Ghosh a lift home and been out to dinner with her and her husband. She reiterated that Dr Harold Heinsson referred patients to his wife from Holloway Prison. "She really dislikes Broadmoor and says it is for detention only, not therapeutic treatment. She complains bitterly of the staff". It still did not sink in how far this antagonism reached and what was happening.

"I don't think the staff like her much but I don't know how anybody can like anybody in these places", I say, "it's moaning about it keeps us cheerful".

My friend continues, "The makers of that film on Ashworth are to make one on Broadmoor – yes, another one – and Chandra wants you to take part". I feel tired. I'm doing a bit of ward work to help out and the school in the mornings. Iris is filling in for me today but, although it's good to be in top gear occasionally I could do with a rest. I cannot get enthusiastic over this film. "If the object is merely to give Chandra Ghosh the opportunity to get back at staff who say they are stopping her allowing some revolting girls do what they want then I'm not very interested", I say part quoting a member of staff. "If professionals can't manage their own system they should not have to rely on patients to do it through TV appearances". Friend listens till I've finished and then says, "Dr Henry Stoll has written to the Home Office complaining you're getting out".

160

Stoll was one of the reasons I was in Broadmoor. I had bonked him quite severely but he had stated forgiveness at the time and not wanted to prosecute. "I wonder", I said, "he's not the one who's paranoid, McNeil is". I had stabbed Dr Desmond Lorne Marcus McNeil in a last ditch attempt to get him to court to give the reason why I had been committed to him back in the 60's. The experience had made me physically ill as well as being a traumatic experience that had left me badly shaken, and I wanted the authorities to understand the counterproductive nature of psychiatry. They would not allow its existence if they knew what it was doing and how it was being manipulated.

Back on the ward it transpires that the notice on the board forbidding patients to visit the rooms of other patients is because of a murder in another "hospital". "There was a pile up on the M4 the other day", I said, "but that doesn't mean the M4 should be closed or motor cars should be banned for ever". This system of dealing with matters, some of which relate to hospitals hundreds of miles away, is the reason that rules get tighter and tighter until someone has to take over to start over again. Alan Franey clearly had a brief to improve Broadmoor. He had a lot of opportunity but the big emphasis through the penal system was to abolish slopping out. To be in a dormitory with no lavatory, only a pot, was to be an experience of the past. To achieve this sanitary improvement, patients at Broadmoor would be able to get up in the night and go to the flush toilet. Bell pushes at a quarter of a million needed to be installed so that staff could be summoned, merely banging on doors to attract attention woke other patients. Then followed personal keys to rooms but staff could override the lock so an inmate could stay locked in if need be. It all took time, a lot of money, a lot of workmen banging away, it did raise the level of containment to the twentieth century but still basic justice and human rights were scarce and needed to be addressed.

The cold bug that has swept through the ward has now got me. For the last two nights in total I've slept five hours waking first with running eyes and then a bunged up nose. I so rarely get a cold that I feel it more when I do get one. Sue S has dodged the ward work. I thought this was because she had the lurgy but Mitch says, "No. She hasn't. She's had a row with her boy friend. It's all off". The boy friend is the ex husband of an ex patient who were the first to hit the headlines with news of their marriage but today's headlines are of Mark Philips' involvement in a paternity suit. It happens in the best families.

Iris has her tribunal (another £650 in legal fees which she can't afford) – and is told she can be transferred to a Dorset clinic. This was recommended by her independent (£250) psychiatrist and unused as Dr Ghosh recommended a hostel. Veronica has her tribunal and the result is her being recommended for transfer to a £180 day hospital – and she wont be coming back here. "Who's paying for you?" we ask, "The District Nurse" says Veronica who keeps giving me Gold Blend coffee. Where has she got it from? Danny says, "It took two doctors to get me here but ten can't get me out". In the news is an acid sprayer who, because no special hospital will have him has got only three years. What politics is being played on this one I cannot imagine. I've not opened my post but must face it first thing tomorrow. I tend to leave official brown envelopes until I feel brave.

It is my birthday, I wear one of the tops my daughter's sent with my friend's cardigan and the "I am 60" badge from the children's cards. The girls unusually did not sing Happy Birthday To You but I had told Sister Irene that I wasn't celebrating because I was still in here. Veronica said I didn't look over twenty, but after protest from me altered this to thirty.

I had a visit. What a carry on. Although my friend arrived at 1.45 the Gate had not called the ward so the escort left without me and I had to wait until more escorts could be found. Luckily there was also a girl from another ward and old Margaret who set up a wail which lasted until we reached the Central Hall. "I don't know who's coming to visit me. I feel awful. I've got no make-up on.   Can you 'old me 'and" and thus we dragged her, me on one side and Nurse Vicky on the other.   There were no visitors for her. The woman on the Gate had "Misread the patients for visitors on the pink form" and a farce had progressed until one visitor had intervened in a conversation with the ward which included, "Her name's Deliah……" "I'm Deliah" she said.   Margaret's sir name is the same as my friend and it was a miracle I had got over there at all.

My friend brought in a four-portion cream and fruit cake concoction which I later smuggle downstairs for Alvada and I to eat between us   I feel obliged to smuggle it as rules come and don't go fast enough and I am not certain if we are allowed to take food with us to another ward without prior consultation.   We sit and do the *Telegraph* crossword despite opposition from TV football and squawks from the record player, which issues its atmospherics if the lid is not down firmly. This ward, which, apart from the parole ward, had been the best on the female wing, was very inconsistent. There was a room at the end of the corridor available as sitting room but sometimes it was occupied by music listeners, whereas our ward had but two noisy day rooms; our highly voluble young element had not tolerated the milk arrangements so on my lesser ward we are issued with a half pint carton each a day whereas on Alvada's nicer ward the women had to scrounge what milk there was left over from the milk jugs at meal times. Their staff took the rest and refused to alter the system. Alvada listens in silence as I tell her about our psychiatrists' staff relationships.

Sue's slacking from ward work has come to a head with Verity's, "I don't work with grassers"; Sue is in seclusion by evening. I go down to see Alvada after lunch and we are munching through some Lymsewold cheese when my name is called. We must not visit downstairs between one and two. News to me. The door between the wards is open but staff must cling onto the last bit of difficulty. I go upstairs and then descend again later to find my friend making salmon sandwiches for Dilly whose nephew is visiting. On my mind is the way correspondence is filed in the Archimedes computer system at school. Alvada is disbelieving when I tell her it is filed under size of letter with no regard to content. "A4 or A5. Take your pick". She is incredulous; I can see her imagining a filing cabinet with items stored according to length of document rather than subject. "A fellow in class the other day did something terribly clever, "she says, "he made swirls of different colours but *I'm* not interested in that are you. That's all right if you're a fabric designer or similar". Computers are new in our lives, we had not yet taken them for granted. All in all, my milestone sixtieth birthday has been pleasant but uneventful. As a child I minded having a birthday that so often fell around Easter. Like a child born at Christmas I was certain that I would have the same number of Easter eggs if I had a birthday in July. I try not to dwell on the brief talk I had with Nurse John who will be on again on Sunday afternoon. He has to write a nursing report on me for HO. I nearly exploded when he told me. Haven't they got past this point yet. Later my Hereford friend tells that it's not the Home Office but SHSA who had also written requesting Chandra Ghosh submit a report. How many times are the same questions being asked by whom and why? The situation is sheer farce. When I ask Bob what the report is for he says he knows nothing about it. He's in charge of the ward and should know what's happening..

Veronica has come down onto the ward and has taken herself into the dining room; suddenly there is an outburst. Veronica is yelled at and ushered out with, "Don't ever come to this ward again" shouted by Sister. At tea Mitch tells me that Veronica had wet herself. She has not been given a promised departure date and yesterday had a couple of fits – the girls say one was fake – and a bout of screaming. Her fits are different from the more usual shaking and falling on floor. Veronica sits rigid and hisses and spits; a recent investigation has discovered "warts on the brain" cause her epilepsy, she says. Ma seems pale and isolated and even plays her squeaky Walkman's at breakfast. She's been in front of the record player all day and seems oblivious to the noise it makes. She's still awaiting a confirmation diagnosis of her weight loss.

Gone With the Wind is on TV, "I don't like those old films" chorus members of the gang at lunch but after tea Iris, Carol – who hasn't seen it previously – and I sit and watch it. I must admit I get more out of it each time round; I saw it first of all at the Watford Gaumont when it first came out and my mother and I took sandwiches to eat in the long interval. "I'm sorry", says the gang member who objected to the film and who has a bump on her forehead from Veronica bashing her with a cup, "but Bob says we can have the video on at 6.30. I think this is a lovely film", she says sinking into a chair and we sigh with relief. "I don't give a damn" says Clark Gable, "Tomorrow is another day" says Vivien Leigh into the sunset. A horror video follows.

On Sunday Scotty retires to bed after breakfast and reappears after lunch; she is suffering from a rejected love affair. John takes a crowd into the garden and I wonder when he'll get round to seeing me to make the report. I decide what I'll do for the Koestler radio play entry but unsure where to start the tale. *Sunday Express* carries the story of Julie Thompson who's been struck off the medical nursing register for spraying an aerosol into the face of a Broadmoor patient. The ward is united that there are far worse than Julie T, who we had found most pleasant, and are belligerent that nothing is done about them. Nurse John sees me briefly about his report but is vague what it's for. I go downstairs to see Alvada and I tell her John says there was an article in yesterday's *Guardian*, which slates Broadmoor. She is not interested. "It won't make any difference," she says. The hour went off last night and I'm feeling it.

There's an announcement that Graham Greene has died aged eighty-six. "Who's he?" says Carol. When I tell her he wrote *The Third Man* she says, "Never heard of it". "It's because you're Welsh" I tease. She's a timid girl who was attacked in the day room for no reason whatever by members of the young thug gang, which illustrated how the ward had become. They punched her and pulled out handfuls of hair leaving a bald patch. Sister Irene decreed that the staff could do nothing about the incident, or punish the attackers, as there were no witnesses. It took a lot of reasoning to see that Carol would constitute no danger to anybody but this way the gang would think Sister Irene was "all right" and not go for her and Carol would feel even more insecure and be more malleable than ever. It's how ward rule is operated.

The MO sees me and organises an X-ray as I spat blood a week back. "It's not because he intends disproving my claims and writing in my files that this is one more illness I've invented", I tell Alvada, "but because he wants to see I'm better". How cynical I have become.

I could still hear Sister Sue say excitedly on the telephone, "He's Gone. We're rid of him". It confirmed rumours that Dr Patrick McGrath, hands-on Medical Superintendent of Broadmoor for a quarter of a century, had retired. He had seen me when I first arrived and removed the medication prescribed by Dr Levin. It was previously maintained that Dr McGrath could not afford to retire, he had "too many irons in the fire" but what this entailed was never explained. It was the end of an era. The end of the extravagant social functions, the monthly male parole dances for some of the most notorious men in Broadmoor. The women were allowed to attend and stay up late till ten o'clock after dancing dressed to the nines to an outside band and eat chicken and chips. Staff could attend in the role of escort for 50p and bring a friend. There seemed no shortage of staff willing thus to spend their free time. Men who never made it past the back wards did not enjoy this lifestyle. It was the start of the end of the overcrowding, which had probably precipitated the emphasis on social functions. It was the end of transparently gross pilferage.

In nearly thirty working years I had never met such an attitude of those in charge as existed in mental hospitals. At Friern Barnet the story told was of six hundred pairs of missing sheets, the culprit saying, "You prosecute me and I'll rat on the rest"; a friend who worked as a secretary at Springfield had to lock up her electric typewriter at night; at Broadmoor the stories rolled. Two generators had "gone missing". Generators! One of the most frequently related tales was of the then Catering Manager, a man called Dibbins, who, when caught trying to fit a side of bacon into the back of his car reputedly threatened the same as the sheet-stealer at Friern Barnet. My Uncle Nom acquired meat on the black market but he paid for it. There is a difference. The attitude was underlined when a male patient had an article censored from the *Broadmoor Chronicle*, the patient's magazine. He had written about a consignment of good quality meat that had been signed for. A while later the meat was collected and cheaper cuts deposited instead. Dr McGrath's comment on the incident was, "One expects it in these places" yet management and staff "in these places" should set a good example to others.

Like most ends to most eras the changeover takes some adjustment. *The Times* had a leading article on the subject of a successor to Dr Patrick McGrath. It read that none of the psychiatrists in Broadmoor were fit to rule. It was apparent to us at Broadmoor that all were still employed; Dr Udwin, renowned for saying that training in social skills "taught rapists to say please" and allowing out three murderers who soon re-offended, would be Acting Medical Superintendent. The *Express* carried a cartoon reading: "Kind Dr Udwin letting psychopaths out of Broadmoor and kind Willie Whitelaw (Home Secretary) letting murderers out of prison.

CHAPTER 8 - BUSHEY

The Post-War Years

I was fourteen in 1945 when peace was declared. We celebrated VE day across the road at the Fitz's; hard-saved rations were produced, where the liquor came from I do not know. There were several families including new neighbours who had married on his day's leave and her afternoon shift off from a factory, the small bungalow flowed with people. On the turntable Joe Loss's *In the Mood* was played over and over again; it was the second record, the first wore out. For a laugh Charlie Chaplin's *Limelight* was put on, the lights dimmed, and Uncle Leo shuffled in with carpet slippers on his knees, wearing bowler hat and carrying a cane. We laughed at his impersonation of Chaplin as Toulouse Lautrec. Everyone was happy. As the clock struck midnight my mother tipsily said it was her birthday, 9th May, and the festivities started again. How naïve of me, of so many of us, to believe that with the war against Germany over everything would return to normal next day. I was too young and innocent to realise that war bred war, peace treaties did not please everyone and previous allies could become bitter enemies. The war in the East went on till August and we cheered in delight when Japan capitulated because America, on President Harry Truman's authority, dropped the first atomic bombs on Hiroshima and Nagasaki. If the war had continued even a few more months many of the prisoners of war who were dying from starvation and malaria in Japanese camps would not have survived. The films of them shown in the cinemas were as bad as those of Belsen and Buchenwald and the stories of torture and deprivation sometimes worse than those of the European concentration camps.   Whereas the Germans ultimately paid compensation to the Jewish people the Japanese resisted paying out and ultimately agreed on a derisory £1.50 per person.   We would never have believed the protest that would result, the Ban the Bomb marches of the sixties the criticism of those who dropped the bomb. For those of us at the time we were delighted that the most ghastly war years of all time had come to an end by whatever means.

For the VJ celebrations Mother and Aunty Joyce went to London and joined the throngs while my father and I stayed at home and bashed the air-raid shelter to bits with sledgehammers. I had hoped Pops would consent to having a pond which would be useful for watering the long garden, too long for our hose pipes, but "they're a nuisance" he said and we bashed away to fill the hole in.

Peacetime brought headline horrors with D (isplaced) P (ersons) Camps for concentration camp survivors who had nowhere to go and no country wanted them. In later years mental hospitals were likened to such places the main difference being that the camps had been inaugurated to work people to death to the benefit of German industry; mental hospitals became places where the inmates provided employment for those who would otherwise have no work.   There was another similarity as every society has those another section of it can do without. In Gestapo Germany criminals were convicted by a court, those taken to concentration or labour camps did not require this legality in the same way that those committed under the Mental Health Act do not require court approval. It became routine for the SS to wait outside a prison for a released prisoner who was not wanted in the community and transport to a labour camp. In the UK it is not uncommon for those in prison to be transferred to top security or other mental hospitals in order that the length of their detention be extended.

Cessation of hostilities brought even more shortages. Bread had not been rationed throughout the war but it was after peace was declared. The delight of sparrows pecking at a loaf of bread, delivered by the roundsman and left on the windowsill, leaving the remains in the middle of the lawn became a nightmare. Pops had run his car frugally throughout the war but had to put it on jacks for a couple of years as petrol became even more precious. He blamed it on the Labour Party and talked about emigrating. My mother went to the cinema the day sweets came off ration in 1951. "I couldn't hear a word for the rustling of sweet papers", she said. The postman still came several times a day and it was still possible to write a letter in the morning and have a reply by the afternoon.

The horror materialised of what had happened to Brenda, the daughter of Aunty Rose to whom I had been evacuated in Devonshire in 1939. Aunty Rose had died of cancer, Brenda staying in the house alone with her mother's corpse for three weeks, let alone the weeks prior to her death, had been found suffering from malnutrition and taken into care. It was a fluke that a social worker, friend of Aunty Winnie Coleman, had recognised the name Wilcox as she met a group of children being transferred across Birmingham. Brenda resembled her father who the social worker had met. The family were horrified that nobody had contacted them; the ease with which my parents had dumped me to safety with Rose and the lack of interest ever since was not mentioned aloud but a sense of guilt was obvious. Brenda's aunt, her father's sister who was my father's cousin, was contacted in Amsterdam through the Red Cross and, as soon as the war was over, Aunty Ethel came over from Holland and took Brenda back there to live.

Aunty Ethel was a story in her own right. She had been a teacher "wedded to her profession", resigned she would never marry who went on an exchange with a South African teacher in 1928. It was the same Dutch captain of the ship that took her there and back and they married. She learnt to speak Dutch and spoke it so well that the Netherlanders complimented her on her English. During the war her husband, Wilhelm, had been obliged to sail with German military on board while Ethel had been an active member of the Resistance, hiding people in her attic. There was a search one night, my cousin Mary was then aged seven and asleep upstairs when the Germans came. The men had stumped up the steep stairs when the officer wandered into the lounge, and said, "You have a German piano".

"Yes", Aunty Ethel replied, "the Germans make good pianos".

"You play", said the officer.

"Yes", said Ethel clutching her dressing gown round her more tightly.

"Play for me" said the man and she did. She played a Beethoven sonata.

"It's all right" shouted the officer to his men upstairs, "there's nothing here". There were people in the loft.

She later severed all contact with this country in disgust at the treatment Brenda had endured and the

Home Office refusal of a work permit for her own daughter Mary. It was my first knowledge of Social Services and their impact. Many years later I understood that Brenda has been slightly spastic and, if kept in care in the UK would undoubtedly have been transferred to a mental hospital to spend the rest of her life. In Holland, she learnt Dutch and ultimately became Assistant Matron of an old people's home in The Hague.

I passed School Certificate with six credits and a distinction in history thereby attaining what was called a Matriculation Exemption. I failed French oral, which did not appear on the certificate to spoil the picture. To this day I can recite Archimedes principle, "When a solid is immersed in a fluid ....." I think I was lucky with the history questions; we had a lovely textbook complete with *Punch* cartoons of the time and written in language I could appreciate - "Napoleon showed his love of law and order by becoming a policeman in the Special Constabulary and his love of humanity by becoming the darling of the ballet girls". Pity I didn't appreciate that this did not refer to Napoleon Bonaparte but Napoleon III but maybe the history paper had not been explicit which one it referred to when asking to what did we attribute the downfall of Napoleon. Too much enjoyment, I wrote. I was rather like the little girl at my mother's school who, when asked to write out the parable of the talents muddled it with that of the virgins. Thus her essay, which stayed pinned on the teachers' staff room board for many years read: "One man buried his, another did business with it and it multiplied accordingly. The master came home and said, 'my good and trusted servant, well done'. English literature was a similar near escape. The set books for London University

School Certificate English circa 1946 included Pope's *Essay on Man*; two days before the exam my poetry-loving mother realised I couldn't understand a word of it. "The study of mankind is man" stuff was not my thing so she rushed to the library and got a copy of *Jane Eyre* also on the list. I read it at one sitting the night before the exam and sailed through. Even at that age I thought it odd that Mr Rochester could marry his first wife and she end up a raving lunatic. What had happened to her I thought.

For the entire stay at Watford Grammar I lived for the year when I could miss the school carol concert and work in the sorting office at Christmas. By the time I was old enough, peace had been declared and these casual jobs went to university graduates home from the war, not schoolgirls. My generation is a cheated one. Born in a depression we are in a minority. When I was eighteen *Vogue Magazine* catered for women of thirty-five. When I was thirty-five *Vogue* featured models in their late teens. On the last day of each term we sang *Jerusalem*, "And did those feet in ancient time....."; I have always loved it.

For everybody, particularly a teenager clothing coupons were a nightmare; nobody would believe me when I refused to stay two more years at school to go to university. "I'm not spending coupons on school uniform any more". I did stay one year for a secretarial course but my father was bitterly disappointed in me despite my arguments that priority for university places was for demobbed servicemen and women and it was unpatriotic to compete with them. Miss Davison, the Headmistress, had me in her office, a nervous-making experience requiring one to gaze at a bulb on the doorframe outside, when it lit up one could enter. She gazed at me and enquired, "I suppose you're going into the Sixth Secretarial because your friends are there". It was not true. I had always had poor handwriting, one teacher had even refused to mark one of my exam papers, and so I resolved to learn to type so others could read what I wrote. I did not argue with Miss Davison, I was too frightened of her to say much and fixed my gaze on her yappy little dog curled in its basket in the corner. Then she fiddled with the papers on her desk and said, "You were quite bright but went to seed although your exam results are quite good". If I had gone to seed at sixteen what would the pronouncement be half a century later.

The peace brought with it the reintroduction of ice cream, withdrawn throughout the war years, and it was not long before Miss Davison stood on her platform at morning assembly to say: "It has come to my notice that girls are frequenting that ice-cream parlour at the back of the market. I must remind you all that it is forbidden to eat in public whilst wearing your school uniform". The uniform was navy blue tunics, or skirts for Sixth Form girls, and pale gold blouses which showed every mark and did not suit those with a sallow complexion. Grillo's was "that place behind the market". They made lovely ice cream.

There was also depression and unemployment as factories switched from munitions to find shortages of raw materials for civilian use. Pops helped me get my first job as a shorthand typist at another Department of Scientific and Industrial Research; by this time he was at Fire Research and I at the Water Pollution Research Laboratory at Watford, which was scheduled to move to a new town called Stevenage. Any hopes I had of being glamorous in my post-school state were short-lived as I had to cycle the six miles to work in all weathers. I decided to get a job in London, which was an even more difficult journey than bicycling. On my first day I knew that this was not for me but had purchased a season ticket. I stayed ten months at the Rootes Group in Piccadilly Circus in an office monopolised by ex WRNS and involving a walk of at least a mile, bus ride on an overcrowded route, and two very packed trains. A man would run ahead of Sir William Rootes when he came round the office and we would hide our handbags and clean up the wastepaper baskets so everything was immaculate. Sir William had a very loud voice and the advance henchman was hardly necessary, we could hear him coming three offices off. Cars for the home market were in short supply, all that could be were exported but there was one man in the office responsible for extracting vehicles for UK VIP's from the production line. His secretary raised her voice so we could all hear her say down the telephone, "Can I always contact you at Buckingham Palace".

Despite the only transport being my bicycle in 1949 I got a job locally. Several members of the tennis club expressed alarm at where I would be working and for whom. "Not him. He's a reputation five miles radius for being an old slave driver." 'He' was a stocky Yorkshire man called Ken Fox who was the Estate Manager and Company Secretary at the Lister Institute, Elstree, where I stayed five years until I married. He always treated me kindly and I admired him enormously

The offices were situated in the Lodge at the end of a tree-lined drive overlooking a kidney-shaped pond and a beautiful cedar of Lebanon; the laboratories were mainly in huts widely situated over the twenty-five acres. There were three of us, the telephonist, me as the shorthand typist and Agatha! Agatha was the bookkeeper, a strict Baptist who did not approve of singing, dancing, the cinema.... She was very jolly to work with! Staff maintained that Mrs Fox had appointed her and Agatha Armstrong stemmed the possibility of being fired by making herself indispensable; she never explained how anything was done or where anything was kept. The joy of her announcement one morning when she handed in a week's notice saying she had been guided by God to join the Lord's Day Observance Society was clouded by the realisation that I would have to do her work until a replacement was found. I had never book-kept. I had no understanding of PAYE. The wages for sixty people (twenty to a page), most working differing hours at varying rates, were calculated on Tuesdays and the total telephoned to head office in Chelsea Bridge Road before 5 p.m. for them to send a cheque to be cashed at the bank on Thursdays. Postal deliveries were then reliable, in five years the valuable cheque never went missing or was delayed in the post.

Although I had a credit in mathematics for School Certificate I still had not been able to balance the wages with the deductions by the time I was supposed to make the telephone call. I wasn't even certain my calculations for 15¾ hours @ 1s.10d per hour (earned by laboratory bottle washers) were accurate, I had nothing to check by. 1s 8d. an hour was easier – there were twelve of those to the pound. There was nobody to ask. Ken Fox's wife ran an animal production farm to supply the laboratory, his eldest son ran a couple of farms and the old man spent as much time at these private concerns as he did at the Lister. He also played golf and went to auctions. The first Tuesday after Agatha departed I was nowhere near balancing the act so I picked up the telephone, dialled the Head Office number and added a hundred pounds to the previous week's total. On Thursday Mr Fox drove me to the Post Office to buy the insurance stamps, postage stamps and savings stamps while he went to the bank. I had learnt how to calculate the number of ten-shilling notes and small change and I added a bit onto each for good measure so we weren't short. After we had finished counting out the money into the wage packets there was a mound of cash in the middle of the table. "We seem to have a very large float Miss Coleman", he said.

"I couldn't add up the figures and get the same total twice running" I said expecting instant dismissal or at the very least an explosion of wrath.

"Oh my God", he replied. "I am sorry. I should have realised. I'll add them up for you" he said and I adored him from that moment onwards although the relief from being offered help to balance the books was rather offset for the moment by the smell of the farm labourers as they came to collect their pay. They looked after the horses required for serum production and the smell of horse manure carried with them was rather strong.

For the next few weeks Mr Fox would make a point of calling in to the office during the late afternoon and balancing the figures for me; he stopped this routine when there were changes in the tax system and he lost his temper over the telephone which he slammed down in disgust as a person at St Albans Inland Revenue explained to him how to make the adjustments. From that moment I had to cope alone.

There were few applicants for the post of bookkeeper and those who were taken on did not stay long. "It's in the middle of nowhere" they would say but we did finish at 5 p.m. and I was so much better off not having to pay fares to London or dress to the nines. Aunty Hap who lived next door (Alf had been evacuated and never returned to her) understood bookkeeping and gave me a *Ready Reckoner*, which became my bible. This was before the days of pocket calculators and adding-up machines had still to become commonplace.

After I passed my driving test the estate maintenance man, Joe, would sometimes let me drive his car home. He had a 1927 Armstrong Sidley with pre-selector gears. The driving wheel had a lot of play, it would not pass an MOT today, and the shock of the clutch riding up as we rode along the Watford By-Pass, produced a "Ppput yorrr bleeding foot on it" stutter from Joe. Some of Joe's several children had passed through my mother's hands at school, she knew them well.

The Lister made all the smallpox vaccine for the country and supplied the armed forces at a penny (1d) a dose. On this relied the profit to fund research. For the production of lymph vaccine two sheep a week were required leaving the carcass intact. Hugh Green was required to kill the animals, which he did for years by knocking them on the head with a sledgehammer. Death was instantaneous but new regulations demanded that slaughter be by a humane killer, which required a gun licence. The first time he used it Hughie nearly shot his thumb off and the sheep were frightened alarmingly. Meat rationing was still tough so the carcasses were cut up into joints on the premises by old Hughie and distributed at four pence

(4d) to staff, threepence for the paper it was wrapped in and a penny for Hugh's time. I was put on the list and received a different cut each week on Tuesdays. Sometimes the parcel would contain offal, sometimes an entire leg. My mother would stand on the doorstep waiting for me as I cycled home, "What have you got?" she would say. It says plenty that this weekly supplement to our meat ration should play such an important part in our lives but my parents had no qualms about eating it. I refused to touch it. I swore, imagined, I could taste the flavour of the vaccine but my mother was so delighted with the gift that she happily donated me both her and my father's meat ration and they ate Lister mutton every week.

At times of food and mouth disease movement licences would be required for the sheep but Mr Fox always dealt with those and the alcohol licence and the man from the Customs and Excise who would call and check if it was kept in the safe and so on. I took odd telephone calls such as the man from the Crown Agents who wanted to place a tender for gonorrhoea antitoxin. He sounded a bit embarrassed. I was nineteen. "Oh" I said cheerfully, "it's obsolete. It's been replaced with penicillin". The Lister was probably unique in the drug industry for never jumping at a sale of anything if the product had been superseded by a competitor's product.

As it contained chlorine the horse carcasses went for pet food. All the horses were named according to when they were purchased, thus those beginning with the letter 'A' could have been purchased in July, the alphabet running out in twenty six weeks to the calendar's twelve months. It was strangely difficult to balance the horses; it would seem a simple exercise to log when one was bought and when it died and how many there were in stock. We spent two hours trying to trace Xinia.

It was custom for the workforce to be vaccinated or tetanus injected, depending on location; but I steadfastly refused any of it, which meant I could roam the grounds but not go into the laboratories that had closed windows. I restricted my holidays to those countries not requiring jabs.

It was at the Lister that I first encountered price fixing in the drug industry. My boss had been trying unsuccessfully for years, through its agents Allen & Hanbury's, to supply tetanus antitoxin to UK hospitals. It supplied against tender to the Crown Agents and exported thousands of doses at around sixpence (6d) a dose. Out of the blue a tender form arrived from a Birmingham hospital and the Lister won its bid to supply in phials three times the price it supplied to the Crown Agents in bulk. From then flowed more tenders from other hospitals when the point was reached that there was a plea from the packing department that they could not cope with the demand. (Packing women earned 1s.8d per hour, a twelfth of a pound). That, however, was a minor problem compared to the telephone call I took where a pharmacist said a patient had died and he had a ward of ill people from tetanus injections. No other hospital had reported problems and, after much testing and retesting it was said to be the solution used to sterilise the rubber caps, not the serum that was at fault. (The serum was bottled so that a syringe was inserted through the rubber cap to draw out the fluid).

The flow of tenders and orders continued until the day arrived when the competitors, Burroughs Welcome and Evans, entered the scene. They summoned my boss to a meeting in Euston Road where it was explained that, for the purposes of distributing tetanus antitoxin, the country was carved in two to supply the product at 2s.6d.a dose. The Lister could be included provided it, too, supplied at this price. The Lister Institute for Preventive Medicine was a non-profit making organisation, strapped for cash, their offices were shabby, their employees paid according to the Whitley Council Scale recommendations – (I was paid a year older than my age group to give me a few shillings extra). The Lister could not participate in such an arrangement, it was against its ethics, but was unable to say so. Mr Fox went missing for a while – his house in Norfolk was hanging over a cliff due to the floods there - and I had to be let in on the situation to man the phone.

After the war neighbours with whom we had been so friendly showed their greater affluence by moving to more expensive areas and eventually my parents acquired a plot of land on the Heath and had a house built. It was a traumatic experience. My mother did not approve the architect's plans, for a start his junior had drawn the lavatory in a room twelve feet long and a yard wide. Typically my mother changed her mind continually on the accommodation she required. In the end my father drew up plans to the latest of her specifications, the builder's brother redrew them to be passed by Town Planning. The builder went bankrupt. All the timber licence was spent on the roof leaving no wood for the stairs, doors or window ledges.....we camped at the Fitz's new house for some weeks with our furniture hoisted up a ladder and stored in the one upstairs room with a door that could be locked. "It's the easiest move we've ever 'ad", said the removal men. My mother was in tears. My father confronted the spiv who appeared, in large car with peroxide blonde companion, who had loaned the builder money to complete the house. The loan shark grumpily surveyed the property, "Told me it was finished that 'arriman did. That ain't bleedin' finished. And said there was val'able trees. Thems sycamores" (he pronounced them sick ee moors), "ain't no good sycamores. Can't bleedin' go and watch me dog run this arternoon". He went on and on. My parents were out of pocket too. The money had been spent by the building labourers playing pitch and toss on the floor instead of working.

It was a lovely house when completed and must have the best post war roof in England. With only a third of an acre my father was delighted not to feel obliged to grow vegetables and my mother equally pleased not to have to look at them growing. She preferred flowers and plain lawn. She continued to teach, this time not for the war but her pension and to continue the argument for equal pay for men and women. She had been upset at being transferred from the boys' to girls' school further up Merry Hill Road. "Girls are so silly", she maintained, "boys are far more interesting"; if ever I needed confirmation that both parents would have preferred a son this was it but the idea of staying at home and reverting to being solely a housewife was not in my mother's nature. She could cook in a very traditional English fashion but more from the necessity of having to eat than fun; she employed a flow of charwomen to do the housework; her sewing was such that she had paid Joyce a packet of cigarettes to finish a dress pinned together on the paper pattern so long the pins had gone rusty and we ate out whenever possible. It took my seeing other families at close quarters to realise that although our cuisine was never venturous it was adequate and even very sparse rations made to last until the next issue. We never ran out of tea or sugar however small the allowance and we always had jam to put on our bread.

CHAPTER 9 - BROADMOOR

Differences of Opinion

The Hereford probation officer, Joe, comes and shows me the report he has written about me. I am described as having undergone a breakdown due to family stress instead of being upset by unwarranted committals. If this is how someone depicts me whose sympathetic attitude is undoubted, then how am I described by those who are hostile? Joe looks drawn and much thinner than when I last saw him.

I have a visit from an old lady who visited another woman in the afternoon. I hope I have that much stamina when I am heading for eighty if I last that long. Civilised visit. Genteel. Escort Shirley is knocking on my door at lunchtime saying Les has nobody at school and where am I. Difficult. I must stop my friend coming in next Tuesday, I can't be in two places at once.

The photos from Princess Di's visit are on show downstairs, £5 a go. Lucky I'm not in them. Mitch and Iris receive accounts from their solicitors for their tribunals. 15% VAT is added. In my room I note that the drawers in my Argos table have been changed over and don't quite slot in; some rough notes I made of Joe's visit have gone from my room during the afternoon. One of the improvements Alan Franey as Chief Executive was to make was the introduction of door keys so we could each open and lock the room to our door with staff keys over-riding. But that hadn't happened yet. For the time being I was thus left wondering if this was an official, or semi-official search or some patient had wandered in. What else was missing.

At school it struck me as funny that all the typewriters and the office computer itself were required to be locked away over the lunch hour and at night whereas the ones in the classroom stayed out. Where else could this happen. Les comes in with the news that the Chief Executive, Alan Franey has suggested that in future there should be a ceremony in the Central Hall to present the exam certificates. Bun fights were what Broadmoor did best but this was clearly recognition that the Education Centre was achieving good results.

The year after I arrived was the Royal Silver Jubilee, which Broadmoor celebrated loyally, although a week after the rest of the country as Jimmy Savile could not attend functions outside and in simultaneously. There had been barbecues not just for every house but down on the Sports Field as well, each event sporting a whole pig and baron of beef with lovely salads and ice cream. By the time of the Golden Jubilee Broadmoor's barbecues were down to one sausage and beef burger. If we could get something going with exam results hey ho for learning.

Back on the ward Debbie tells me that Alvada had come up to see me this afternoon. Ah ha. I thought. Have Joe's notes turned up again. I go and look. Yes. They have. Alvada has a naughty streak. I had met this particular trait in her before, actually seen her in my room rifling through a file when she thought I was in the bath and I had been stupid enough to tell a member of staff. I had been moved to the ward downstairs where I should have been years previously but for some reason had been overlooked. It was then much better downstairs with the rooms unlocked all day whereas York II had them locked. The snag to it was that I jumped the queue, avoided the dormitory and was given a decent room and the girl who had to wait longer in the dormitory was spiteful and vengeful. Over the years Alvada had been promoted and I moved back up because of my ears. This somewhat circular movement reflected progress at Broadmoor but at the time I had found her in my room going through my belongings when she thought I was in the bath, Alvada was put on medication. I felt terrible seeing her shaking and hobbling on Depixol and the experience taught me never to go to the staff again about another patient, however much troubled me. I never understood what Alvada thought I was writing but I was one of the few people who could comprehend the anguish caused at what had happened to her and I thought any mention I made of her displayed the sympathy I felt for her having her insides wrenched out needlessly. Hysterectomies had become the vogue. I remember seeing a gynaecologist at University College Hospital who had informed me he could do one on me, "What do you want it for?" he had said. I lay on the bed thinking, "Why don't you have yours off. What do you want yours for?" but I was very polite, stayed mute but fled back to my GP and asked for another referral where I was made better by a mere d & c. Most upsetting was my cousin Jill with whom I had been evacuated years ago. She had contracted cancer; a few weeks before she died the surgeon removed her ovaries "to prevent the spread of infection", the infection had already spread to her major organs and she was patently dying. She minded terribly and her family, me too, were most upset that her last days were made

188

more horrid than need be.   A feeling of impotence in the face of the dire, when no help is possible, is sickening but it is better to do nothing than make the inevitable worse.

On the phone my daughter tells me that my grandson has completed only two of the twenty arithmetic books at school; he's bored doing childish sums.   He resembles his maternal grandfather, my ex husband, and I wonder if tomorrow's visit to the headmaster will earn spanking or sympathy.

Alvada comes upstairs and is intent on questioning me about my friend in Hereford. How did we meet and so on. I gather she is inferring, without letting me know she's read it, that Joe's report is influenced by misinformation passed by my friend and not the distorted "medical" reports I blame it on and the desire by all in the system to defend it.   Yesterday she had inferred that Princess Di visited Broadmoor because of her, Alvada. The staff would be concerned. writing copious notes and upping her medication if they knew so I ignored it. The mood would blow over. It only needed something to cheer her up.   We are handed our census forms – special abridged ones for those "in care". I stated that I am incapacitated due to MHA committal although sane. I do not doubt that others did similar or that the censors took no notice and our observations were unrecorded.

Oh dear. I'm making such a mess of the school job. I can only be fired. I type a list; it prints one side of the central heading with just a few letters appearing on the left hand side. Dan is in the library, helpful as ever but can't see how to fix this one. I try again.   The escort staff are yelling for me, "Come on" before I've finished another memo. I worry that I've corrupted the file. Have I Quit properly. Keith, another inmate, who makes the teas will lock up for me and is looking at me more and more pityingly. Computer systems have improved since then but that was no comfort at the time. I worried all weekend. Back on the ward I play Scrabble with Carrie and calm down a bit. I wonder how my grandson faired with his headmaster. Can he or can't he do his sums. Is he now truculent or smiling.

Mitch won't say which days she leaving but is upset that two sisters and one other are taking her to the hostel. This is an excessive escort by any standards particularly when being "discharged into the community". She worries if there'll be room left over for her belongings, stereo and so on in the vehicle taking her.   "Oh we can send them on later in the week" says Nurse Bob cheerfully – whether to console or rile her nobody can see. It is surprising how much people accumulate in a small room over the years. She's now been told that Bob won't be going with her, he's on duty then, so SNO Lenny Dunn is going. "What on earth for?" we ask.   Staff go on escort when off duty, on overtime.

I see a duty doctor over my hobbling foot. He's diagnosed arthritis. I feel ninety. Eug is partially up from seclusion after her smashing episode but obsessive that the wrong TV is on. The smoking room has ITV and the non-smoking BBC and they're both showing ITV. At lunch Sister Irene displays paranoia and insists that only one table at a time should get up and go to the hatch to be served, "In case there's a disturbance and we have to call staff over". In case of disturbance I doubt many of us would remain seated at our tables waiting patiently for the alarm bell to be rung while plates and chairs crashed onto us before being rescued by male staff thundering in.   Sister Irene was clearly exercising her imagination and I could see she was nervous of Eug who is a tall Afro-Caribbean of no mean strength. Irene is a short Afro-Caribbean. Things can change but Eug is like a volcano, erupting rarely, in her case not more than once every three or four years but causing chaos if the warning signals are not spotted in time to evacuate.

After lunch there is a ward meeting. Unkind of us to remark to each other that there is no Senior Nursing Officer or doctor present. Julie is upset that her vibrator has been taken off her. She was allowed to have it, the purchase authorised by the ward psychiatrist and other members of the Clinical Team and a subject of ribald humour all over Broadmoor; the transport manager (male) had been out to buy it and now she didn't have it. The Staff didn't think it was suitable. It was a risk item. "I'm going to sue Broadmoor for the cost of it", Julie cries to our howls of amusement.

I watch the news in the corridor on Ma's miniature TV plugged into a wall socket. We have a computer on the ward and Sister Sue shows me how to play with it. It's a primitive gadget compared to the ones at school but quite fun. A resident announces she's to go to Heatherwood Hospital to have the plates in her mouth removed as she's had a mouth infection and lived on antibiotics ever since her jaw op.   She did not know she had any plates in at all.

Viewing is no-good-to-go-to-bed-on.   Documentary on our prisons – horrendous. What has this country become. At least they're not as bad as Bolivian or North Korean ones. At 8.30 Nurse Mary asks me to give June her laundry. The rest of the ward drew theirs at 5.30. As I need Nurse Mary to unlock a door and cupboard I wonder why Nurse Mary does not handle the matter herself without calling me to actually extract the items from the shelves. I do not feel valued and needed. The sheets were all stamped, "Broadmoor Hospital" but on one occasion I found one marked, "Mortuary" which I promptly handed to a nurse.

Debby had also drawn no laundry. She had slept with coverless duvet and no pillowcases. Lack of towels did not bother her but then washing is not a strong point either. Veronica departs in true style for her private hospital in Hertfordshire. Screams of, "I want to f...g see what I'm wearin'" and demands of the staff to open her door so she can see her "f....g" coat. A remark that her coat was not indulging in sexual exercise produced even more screaming. I turn off my light to be bellowed at by Eug who is out of seclusion during the day, "Don't you turn my light off" followed by, "You've tried to kill me twice. You'll never get out you evil old woman". I shout an apology for turning off the wrong switch from the panel in the corridor. Later Mitch tells me she's had the same barracking. Kathy is late for lunch and asks Ma about ECT. I am shocked, Kathy is shaky and very insecure but that's the environment and the drugs and the reason that brought her here. ECT will not cure the past. Later in the day Kathy is taken to the Block. Mitch, Ma and I all agree that this is very odd. There are far worse than Kathy on the ward who killed her child when the father of it brought his latest girl friend to her flat and had sex on the sofa in front of her. Sue has eaten glass, we're told. From the Stores on the ward I get the tapestry I'm doing for the Koestler Award. Can I do a small picture in three days, the closing date is nigh. I'm embroidering a view of Broadmoor through the window bars, more interesting than a heraldic shield, which is another category. I'm still hobbling but don't like to think about it. I gather my lungs are intact, the blood spitting not explained.

I finally meet Mark, the young author who's coming in to take a Creative Writing course. Les really does his best to fill the needs of a wide variety of inmates and creative writing is a new innovation. The Broadhumourist had produced Alan Ayckbourn's *Confusion*, which had been showing twice a week for a couple of months before the final show for the patients. It was very good and we all barracked and clapped at the wrong moments. This would be followed in a few weeks by a Green Room Dance to which the cast invited other patients to attend and have a mixed grill supper. I went several times but not this time, the fellow who used to invite me had been transferred. Proceeds, frequently over a thousand pounds and rising, from the Broadhumourists went to nominated charities. It cost three times the amount collected to fund the staff escort required for rehearsals and the actual showing to the public but it was not popular to mention this.

Another innovation at the school was a series of meteorological lectures and a University lecturer came in from Reading. He stared at Alvada open mouthed when she remarked in her American accent why weather forecasts mattered in England as the weather was always so predictable. As an after dinner gambit this was lovely but it was not appreciated by the Man

193

from the Met. This was the week there were thirty hurricanes, l00 metres diameter, across Kansas, Alvada's home state. Bangladesh had a cyclone of 500 meters diameter in which an estimated 50,000 people died and twenty million made homeless; we feel small and insignificant. The elements are bigger than even the POA. (Prison Officers Association).

Fran visits with the baby who entertains all in the Central Hall; she is very demanding and lively unless played with constantly. It was a lovely visit and helped take my mind off Dr Ghosh's report, which raised my blood pressure and left me feeling helpless. What can I do? I'm never going to get out with this report. At school Bill C had commented that the reports for a tribunal on him were "Like a death warrant". What gets into those in authority that they paint such rosy pictures of those who are law abiding under normal circumstances but make no allowance when the circumstances for others are abnormally intolerable. Who was it that wrote, "When injustice becomes law resistance becomes duty?". I felt very dutiful.

The Spring Holiday was cold, more like an autumn break. The next event at school was Dr Murray Cox's lecture on Shakespeare's plays for which I managed to produce a classic computer error in the poster advertising it. The print emerged double the size on one side of the paper and half size on the next line. Neither Tutors Ann nor Mike knew how I had achieved this. It merely added to my worries. I keep thinking about the piffle the question and answer stuff between SHSA and Broadmoor really is, a telephone call would clarify the reason I was on no medication and so on. It was clearly a time-wasting exercise, the papers had not gone to the Home Office and I doubted they ever would. Even if they did I understood that Parliamentary Under Secretaries were apt to ignore the pile of release notices to be signed and concentrate on unsullying their careers by not allowing a dubious person to go. Lower down the scale the Mecca of those at the Home Office was the Foreign Office and they stood no chance of a transfer there if they had made a wrong decision at HO. I had read an article in a newspaper headed: **Disaster at the Foreign Office. 'It was an extension of the bureaucrat's fervent belief that if you do nothing, then, miraculously, nothing will happen** and it seemed that those at the Home Office had adopted the same attitude; SHSA followed suit. It was miraculous that anybody was released at all.

Greenlanders seemed far more sensible; with twenty-five thousand miles of coastline there isn't a single prison. There is the usual range of crime, murder, rape, larceny and so on and there are law courts but the idea of retribution is unknown. Only psychopaths are shipped off to Denmark for detention, the most an "ordinary" murderer can expect is to be required to sleep in a special house each night for, say, five years during which time he can carry on working, visit friends and family during the day but he is quite likely to be ostracized by those who disapprove of his crime. Being sent to Coventry can make life difficult and work impossible but that is another issue. This country is too entrenched in its traditions of drawing and quartering its enemies and transporting its deviants to the Colonies which makes the solving of social problems, a root cause of so much violence and emotional disturbance, something to be deferred to another day. I did not know then that the Chief

195

Executive at Broadmoor and that at SHSA had been appointed to either improve special hospitals or close them. All I could see was that the formation of SHSA provided one more handicap for patients to overcome, one more blockage to release, a change of badge on the caps of male staff and a furtherance of the jobs for the boys routine. Maybe I'm like Dorothy in the *Wizard of Oz* who found the wizard was really a little man hiding behind a barrier he had erected for his own protection. Is the man with the fountain pen at the ready to sign release forms like that. For some reason I am remembering a journey from Exeter years ago. The train stopped at Reading and a group of men boarded carrying brief cases embossed OHMS. Were they from the Home Office visiting Broadmoor or Reading jail? How little I understood the penal system then Or understand it now for that matter.

My daughter's letter says my granddaughter is to go to proper school in September when she will be four years three months. It seems very early. Her brother was not allowed in until five and a quarter and then held back and is so bored. Inconsistent difficulties start at an early age.

This time I can blame the weather for a restless night as much as the torch-flashing staff. I have jammed the sash windows down the corridor and in my room with paper towels, which, in the interests of security, are soon removed and inspected in case there is anything wrapped inside.

The day has dawned for Dr Murray Cox's lecture on Shakespeare's plays. The classroom is full; it is raining outside and the speaker makes a theatrical entrance waving umbrella and shaking wet mackintosh. We were handed some photocopies of the first pages of *King Lear,* "The storm. The storm", sighs our lecturer who proceeded to show us video clips of famous actors who had played the lead. He then regaled us with imitations of how a cigarette could be used theatrically and it was plain that he had performed thus for many a dinner party. "When a rapist says 'Oh I didn't mean to kill her'" we understood that Broadmoor patients are frequently discussed and mimicked. As a discourse on Shakespeare's plays the lecture was a dismal failure – we did not get past page one – but as a demonstration of an analyst preparing for the next dinner party he was amusing. He was married to Baroness Cox, Deputy Leader of the House of Lords under Margaret Thatcher, and we always assumed the slanting of the Mental Health Act (Amendments) 1983 was due to marital influence.

Another well-attended lecture was one Saturday morning – the Education Centre operated only five days a week and a couple of evenings but the enthusiasm concerning it allowed more flexible opening when required – when a young Swiss with a degree in Alfred Hitchcock's films came in. He too had clips of films to show us and had us guessing and discussing which foot kicked first in a scene from *Strangers On A Train*. I puzzled him by saying the one wearing co-respondents shoes must be the criminal. He did not know what the term 'co-respondent' meant and I had to explain this to the innocent gentleman in front of a crowd of men. Les Martin was nearly in tears with laughter as were the rest of the group.

  The physiotherapist is back after losing her father who struggled and fell out of bed in hospital when attached to a drip; he had been in such pain the physio thought he had broken some bones so he was

ninistered morphine which finished him off. It was
e last straw when she got home from the hospital
nd a huge picture of her grandfather fell from the wall
as she opened the door. She looks strained even
now but is helpful about my back and foot. I suffer the
pummelling in the belief that it is helping.

Sisters Irene and Dorothy interview me over the new
"Nursing Process". This time the questions and
answers are on a blue card. How does the patient
view her problems? Objective and methods. How do I
say that SHSA are my latest problem? That is not a
recognized problem. We each had to sign the card to
agree what was written. Although not agreeing I sign
in the knowledge that this latest innovation will be a
nine days wonder, if that, then forgotten and ignored.
Their words, "Does not think she has mental illness"
infers that they do (think I'm bats). "We have to say
that", they say but I can see no reason why that should
be the case but I am too bored to get involved in a
lengthy explanation or argument on the subject. What
is the use of arguing with a wall, a wall that is
frightened of putting its job on the line and speaking
the truth? When I closed the office door I noticed
Dorothy explode in exasperation, yet it is I who should
be exasperated at over-long detention. Three days
ago I was told that Bev is now my Primary Nurse, John
has left to become a prison officer for real, and I've just
had Dorothy, so I really have lost track of who is
supposed to be doing what.

A ward meeting appoints me to get up a petition to
complain at canteen prices. I know, but the others
wont accept it that the canteen is the equivalent of a
corner shop, it is not a supermarket, and no amount of
petitions will alter this. However I do my best and

most people sign what I draw up. Despite this it was a pleasant weekend. At long last I caught up with watching *A Passage to India* and *Butch Cassidy and the Sundance Kid*; I actually saw both films right through. I hope this improvement is prophetic.

Alvada had a visit from Joyce, who used to be here and outside is friendly with another patient, John; he's been given a council flat but at the age of forty two and after twenty odd years in here has no references for a job, so, for very little, programmes for helpless patients at the local mental hospital and helps Joyce with her garden. It seems like a problem the authorities need to take on board and it can't be much fun for John with no prospects of earning a proper living despite being qualified and able to work.

Whilst we're waiting in the canteen Shiela points to a plaque on the wall framed by a blue velvet curtain. "This shop was opened by Andrew McKay MP 20 May 1991". So that was it. That explained why a petition to protest at the prices was suggested and I was conned into the organizing of it. Poor Mr McKay. He too could not have known what he was opening. We became used to the plaques on walls. Virginia Bottomley, then Health Minister, opened the new Education Centre and signed the visitors' book with the pen I handed her – we'd taken some trouble to select the best we had – the Central Hall had one to mark its renovation with swathed curtains and pink-painted pillars by Mark Rylance from the Royal Shakespeare Company; Princess Diana had several.

I witnessed in entirety The Ministerial opening of the Education Centre, which had been in operation for some months before the official ceremony. The plaque was to be placed in the school entrance hall where there was insufficient space for all the visitors to sit so a stand was wheeled into a classroom containing the plaque and curtain to be pulled, there was a company that specialized in hiring this out, delivered it, collected it after the string was pulled and, if required, nailed the plaque to its final resting place. Potted plants fronted the stand holding the plaque. There were looks outs shouting a warning when the entourage were sighted and we all scampered to our positions mine being in my office guarding the Visitors Book and ready to hand over pen. Immediately the ceremony was over and the visitors gone, little men ran in to remove the potted plants to where they were next needed. There was lovely food, the entourage retired to the Central Hall to eat theirs and we learned later the Vicar's wife had been unable to obtain a piece of gateau of which I managed two pieces in the Education Centre.

The news is dominated by the assassination of Rajid Gandhi. *The Times* describes the widow as a plumber's daughter, yet what Italian plumber sends his daughter to Cambridge? *The Telegraph* is more illuminating, it says she is a builder's daughter and happy when conversing with Italian businessmen. If Sonia Gandhi had favoured English businessmen would readers be told she was a director's daughter? Come what may, by lunch time the widow has turned down the offer to lead the Indian Congress Party. What can it be like to be widowed so suddenly and within five minutes be asked to run the same risk?

A hernia explains ma's loss of weight. She is prescribed medicine and on a diet. Dr Ghosh sees me before lunch and mentions I might get a visit from the

TW TV team who have been banned from visiting. It seems I have no choice but I am interested. There have been several TV companies in Broadmoor but none of them hit the spot and say psychiatry is counterproductive as it is a root cause of many of the problems confronted by Special Hospitals. A BBC film did show a male patient asking the camera, "Know what the anagram of psychiatrist is?" " Shitty craps" was the answer.

At the start of Alan Franey's reign as Chief Executive there were several films of Broadmoor and public relations extended to visitors of patients allowed a conducted tour. Heather came in with my daughter and a friend of hers and we sat on the Terrace eating a nice meal topped with pineapple ice cream. By the time Franey left such events were history; by the time Julie Hollyman, a psychiatrist, became Chief Executive, no film crews were allowed in and any footage now shown on television is from reels made in the 80's and early 90's. Probably the only one to make a real impact and have effect was *The Silent Hospital* on Rampton, which did result in improvements of regime but not to the Mental Health Act itself, which is a root cause of much disturbance as it is so unjust.

My friend from Hereford visits with S from TW who has a tape recorder in her handbag, the same as that designed specially by Princess Anne for her meetings. It costs £250. This could not happen today. Visitors are not only required to empty their pockets but leave their handbags behind and go through metal detectors, body searches…only the resolute can face Broadmoor's visiting arrangements today. I can console myself that I did what I could; I never turned down an opportunity like this to deplore the psychiatric system. The three of us sat, my friend mute, while I did most of the chatting with prompts from the reporter. It was hard to start, it always is. It's a long story.

CHAPTER 10 – THE PAST RETOLD FOR THE PRESENT

I lived with my husband and two year old daughter in Hampstead. We were lucky to get the two-bedroom flat near the Heath, which had been built on a bombsite. The original house must have been hit near Christmas – one day when I was digging in the shrubbery at the front I found a bunch of old tallow candles tied together with the remains of red ribbon. However, I had some trouble with my eyes and the GP, Dr Henry Stoll, referred me to the local hospital, The Royal Free. There the Indian locum ophthalmic specialist made passes at me. My problem was that I was polite and totally unused to this sort of behaviour from professionals and I thought I'd dealt with him when I removed his straying hand for the umpteenth time saying, "Do you make passes at all your women patients?".

"Only the pretty ones" he said and we go into a clinch. I should have reported him then and there but I felt pity for an immigrant doctor, didn't wish to cause trouble and was merely polite. I was issued with a prescription for glasses and some eye drops. Three weeks later there's a ring at the front door and there he is. He smilingly tells me he got my address from the hospital file he could not get me out of his mind. He raped me. It's as simple as that. Afterwards he asked me where my husband worked and unwittingly I told him, it was a well-known firm and we were both proud of him being there. That evening John was not only late from work but clearly agitated. His only words were, "I'm driving you insane. I'm driving you insane". He was in another world and I could not talk to him. I was in a terrible state, really frightened at what had happened and now my husband seemed hardly aware of what he was doing or saying. The next day he lunged at me, put his hands round my throat and only my horrified struggling and his breakthrough with sanity saved the day. I phoned a friend of his to say John and I were splitting up, "Another one. You're the third in a fortnight" said the friend and John went to stay with him and his wife who I trusted to look after our little girl with their sons, I to another friend who had a miscarriage the day after I arrived and I looked after her two children, husband and father. John moved out of the flat and I later moved back in with our child who stayed with him and the friends at weekends; I got a job with a local company.

It was then the telephone calls started. John was obviously in a state ranting and shouting, "You'll get what you deserve. I don't envy you what's going to happen to you". I just let him shout it out but it was out of character for him to be so voluble though I recognized he was a slighted Apollo. Then there was another unknown caller who just listened and I put the phone down pretty promptly but I thought it was the eye doctor. Occasionally he would murmur questions how I was and was I alone. Can one identify a person's breathing down the phone with muffled undertones? If you try hard enough you can convince yourself of anything. My mother was the worst. When I told her we'd split up she was absolutely hysterical. What would the neighbours say? She kept ringing and saying, "Tell me. I don't understand". She apparently crawled round the floor being sick and howling so my father came up to London for the day to see me. He told me he was dying of cancer, had six months to live and I should make his last days happy by returning to my husband. I was struck forcibly how my interests in being happy were never the concern of either of my parents. What the neighbours thought ruled. Apart from the idea that was forming in my mind that everyone had gone mad I discovered I was allergic to a flowering shrub in the garden which was the cause of the sore eyes that had got me referred to the eye man. It had been planted some years and only recently started blooming.

A few weeks later, out of the blue, I received a letter from the Middlesex Hospital Psychiatric Department. Psychiatry was fashionable then, the profession had launched a great deal of publicity to advertise its benefits, sex linked to psychosomatic ailments much in evidence, marvellous new cures from wonder drugs and I was intrigued to meet one of these people who seemed to have the answer to the world's ills. I conveniently forgot the girl at school who had been disturbed at her encounter and the couple to whom I had been bridesmaid whose child had been slow to develop. They had been referred to a child psychiatrist in Edgware who had pronounced that the maternal grandmother's presence in the house was the cause of the two year old being unable to stand up or talk. The couple had nearly broken up over the diagnosis until they woke up and asked the GP for another referral. At Great Ormond Street they were informed that the child was severely handicapped, tests showed only half her brain had developed; the parents resolutely refused to have her either used as a guinea pig for students and have deaf parts of her brain removed or put into care and she died at eleven years of age at home. I forgot all this and, knowing nobody else who had seen a psychiatrist, cheerfully kept the appointment wondering what it was all about.

The letter had been strange, the appointment was at lunchtime and stated, "You should take refreshment beforehand as no meal will be provided". I had never heard of any outpatients providing meals. Where had the hospital obtained my name?

At the hospital I was greeted by an incredibly enthusiastic medical student who explained that he would interview me, and then I would see Professor Pond with other students and then the Professor by himself. I quickly surmised that the last interview would be the one with the nitty-gritty; the rest would be to amuse the students. I quickly became tired of the interviewer's eagerness, his broad beaming grin was almost provocative and I could not resist the urge to startle him. Marilyn Monroe once said to a psychiatrist, "You call me mad, OK. I'll act mad" and she removed all her clothes. I know how she felt but I didn't have a body like hers but I d just done the shopping and had a six-pack of lager with me.

"Do you think this is a substitute for mother's milk?" I said brightly producing a bottle, "can you open it for me". The student was clearly nonplussed but I was insistent, "I'm thirsty, I need a drink" and he ultimately took the proffered bottle and used a tap to open it. I did my best to continue to entertain him and he went off to confer with the Professor. I was guided into another room, all the students were grinning widely, their mentor looked suitably serious. He waved a hand for me to be seated; the hand waving seemed a major part of his communication skill, he could not look me in the face, he gazed at a point at least forty-five degrees distant. The Professor had a problem and it was not me. I wondered what his wife was like.

I waited in vain for some kind of apology or explanation for having my time wasted coming to visit him but the questions became more and more impudent and the students grinned wider.

"How is your sex life?", he enquired and I have to admit to a glib reply, "Quantity not quality" which wasn't strictly accurate but seemed to please him. "This problem", he waved but I couldn't recall saying it was a problem. "I'd let you keep your clothes on", he said with another distant gaze, faint smile, and another effeminate flutter. "Er", I managed. At this point I was told to wait outside. I was still trying to work out what was implied by the conversation when the student bustled out, panting with excitement, even more so than previously.

"I'm just going to ring and see which hospital can take you", he said. I waited until he was out of sight and then I ran. I took a taxi home and when I got there I poured myself a huge brandy. That evening I went to see Dr Henry Stoll, my GP.

"The psychiatrist was mad", I said and he looked at me sadly.

"They all are", he replied. Why, if he thought they were mad did he refer me to one? I had to assume that it was he who recommended me. What the blazes was going on; that was the end of it, I thought.

A few weeks went by and then my mother wrote saying, "Take a taxi here", my parents lived in Devonshire, I in London NW3, "before they get you". A cheque was enclosed and the phone calls mounted.

I again visited my GP and enquired, "Could you please tell me what is going on".

"Go home", he said, "and somebody will come and explain it to you". So I went home and after a while the doorbell went, a fellow pushed his foot in the door saying in a Scottish accent, "I'm from the Mental Health Department" and barged in. I was completely flummoxed. I let him use my phone; he did not offer to pay for the call. He called in another man who I later understood to be a Medical Officer. He didn't even speak to me but I understood that I should go with Mr James Baird.

"I've a child at nursery school", I said.

"That'll be taken care of" was the offhand reply and I was stood over as I packed a bag with no idea how long for or what was entailed.

I was bundled into a car and James Baird proceeded to chat. He had been born in a mental hospital, he said, and I assumed his parents worked there. Clearly mental hospitals were his life and his aim to fill them up. "You're not going to Friern Barnet", he chattered, "they had to change the name from Coney Hatch as there were so many music hall jokes about it. I'm taking you to Horton Hospital in Surrey, which is part of the Camden catchment area. There are seven mental hospitals in Epsom as well as the racecourse". I stayed silent most of the time, sick with apprehension. I wondered whether to bound out of the car as we drew up at traffic lights but thought better of it. On arrival at the grim Victorian asylum Baird walked me jauntily down the corridor smiling at the several beggars sitting with hands outstretched for cigarettes. "I've got another one for you", he says as we enter the locked ward, "I'll fill you in on the details".

I was treated like a criminal; my fingerprints and mug shots were taken and I was stripped for an offensive medical supervised by a fishwife Irish nurse. I was very frightened indeed and when I'm scared I either crack jokes or go quiet. I was very quiet. The lavatories stank and were disgusting, the food worse than my memory of wartime school dinners. At my first meal a plate went whizzing past my ear like an UFO, crashed into the wall and the contents slid down in greasy streaks. "I'm not hungry thanks" I said when it was my turn to be served. At bedtime everybody was given night sedation – usually chloral hydrate, "A precaution against gang rape in the dormitory" a patient explained. Separate rooms the experts then maintained, were potentially harmful owing to the increased opportunity to masturbate.

By the time I was led into the psychiatrist the next day I had decided there was very little wrong with most women on the ward; they were a mixture of angry, sad and confused at the treatment they had received. A Nigerian woman maintained her husband had put her there so he could go back home and get another wife. As I walked into his consulting room Dr Desmond Lorne Marcus McNeil stared at me, his fingers poised around a pen. He could have been a blood relative of Professor Pond. "Why am I here?" I asked.

"Why do you think you're here?" says the doctor loftily.

"You must be short of patients", I said not realizing that he would write this down to substantiate my committal. To him his ward was full of mental patients requiring his treatment; to me the ward could be cleared in a couple of weeks by a couple of able secretaries. The main difficulty seemed to be that few women had homes to go to. I learned later that I was labelled paranoid schizophrenic the treatment for which was Stelazine and ECT. All I had needed was a rational explanation why I had been targeted by psychiatry and the part played by the eye man. There were three of us on the ward convinced we were subjects of a community psychiatric exercise; the treatment we received did not make us believe otherwise. I stayed friendly with the other two women for some time and attended the wedding of one of them.

After the first dose of Stelazine my hands went numb. I couldn't feel my fingers. I couldn't keep still and yet I felt sleepy. The shock treatment was given in the dormitory with the feet on the pillow. I was startled at this, as a few weeks earlier I had had a dream. I rarely dreamt so this was a strange occurrence for me. In the dream my head was on a bed where my feet would normally be and a man's voice said, "It's all right. She can take it". In the dream I knew I could not take it but I was unable to speak. In fact I was so withdrawn after ECT that the treatment was stopped after four doses, the normal course is six. On the brighter side I learned that ECT had originally been given without anaesthetic, the holding down of patients frequently causing broken bones. I was appalled that nurses could give such treatment after witnessing the results once and I came to the conclusion that either such personnel lacked a certain insight into the harm they were inflicting or they were sadists. They were frequently likened to personnel in concentration camps obediently doing the job they were detailed to do. I gradually recovered and became acquainted with the other women. The plate-smasher was Jacqueline, aged fifteen, in for care and attention, as her mother could not cope with her at home. She asked me to sew up a hem and, even though there were better needlewomen on the ward than I, she insisted I did it for her. Jacqueline was pregnant by another patient. Would this have occurred if she had been allowed to stay at home? What is care and protection?

My parents visited; my mother was apparently told my incarceration was all her fault and that because of her I would never re-marry. It was at this point she started drinking and never really stopped. She had a low tolerance to alcohol, two gins and she was out, so perhaps the term "drinking" is ambiguous. I was appalled that they drove off and left me, my mother sending another cheque to "get yourself out of there."

I played tennis with another girl and a fellow transferred from Parkhurst acted as ball boy. My self-esteem could not sink lower after the realization that I was in company with convicts. My tennis opponent told me about a recent admission, an American girl. "She was raped by her psychoanalyst in the interests of her analysis and when she told him she was pregnant he refused to see her. After he'd refused to open his door to her she was in tears as she walked down the street and the Police picked her up and brought her here". It transpired that McNeil had contacted her parents, "friends of the Kennedy's" to come and collect her and he had given her something so she was no longer expecting. Although it was prior to the Abortion Act and therefore an illegal act on the part of the psychiatrist, I think this abortion was the only action of his that I agreed with the entire time I was at Horton. How different was the plight of Jacqueline; McNeil sent her to school when she was four months gone; she stayed a day. I was angry at the double standards.

I stayed three months until the psychiatrist's Arab assistant interviewed me and said, "I can't be bothered to renew this section. Pack your things, you can go".

"I can go?", I was stunned. I was insecure in a way I had never previously known, my hands shook from the drugs, I could not even hold a cup to my lips, I had to bend down to the table to drink.

"Yes". I left solely for the reason that I intended to discover why I had been sent to the gruesome place to be sullied and degraded, I felt my life was over, and I could have stayed there until I died. The reason that prompted my going home was the determination to get to the truth. Forever I have the memory of Dr McNeil standing by the office door surveying the women on the ward, many comatose; the superior sneering look on his face said it all.

During the three months of my incarceration in what I called a concentration camp Nicky had settled down with her father who had moved out to a house we were buying in the country. I would now have her alternate weekends. I stayed at the flat but had to earn some money to live on and this prevented me dwelling too much on how dirty I felt; for a long while I bathed twice a day to try to wash away the stench of that disgusting place and I could not rid myself of the feeling that those in authority could have no conception of the mire called mental hospital. The bulk of the people did not need to be there.

The thought of social security never occurred to me. I went to an employment agency and was sent as a temporary to an office in the City where the managing director's secretary had retired suddenly after a heart attack. I seemed to thrive on employers with terrible reputations, this one had earned a reputation of "killing them off", "them", being his secretaries. Like mental patients who demand attention, ignoring them works wonders. I learned from another secretary detailed to show me the ropes that I was one of a long line of temps; my boss when he appeared in time for coffee surveyed me with a mixture of relish and resignation but I was used to difficult men. After a couple of days a smoked salmon was delivered the attached note read: "The prize for getting the least wet". The chauffeur when he appeared to check on the day's itinerary said, "'e won't carry that 'ome. It smells. Give it me, phone his 'ome and tell the gardener to meet the 4.30". Sir said not a word next day but I expected to be dictated a thank you note. I expected in vain so typed a letter with the usual thanks, the last sentence reading, "If this is what I get when someone falls in the river I'll certainly see it happens again". Sir read it, a slow smile spread across his face and he sighed, "You will stay wont you", he murmured, "The pay's quite good". The pay was more than I had dreamt of and it was doubled again within eighteen months.

My trouble was that I could not sleep. The GP gave me a prescription for chloral hydrate and I found that even though I slept with it I would wake up again and I had got into the habit of taking another swig making it very difficult to wake up in the morning. I was haunted by the experience of Horton. If I was considered insane by experts and I was accepted by businessmen what did this mean. My downstairs neighbour who had been severely crippled by childhood polio would phone three rings to wake me, which didn't cost any money, and then give me a lift to Kings Cross each morning. How I would have managed without her I do not know.

I kept the appointment to see McNeil and he was horrified when I told him I had stopped taking the drugs. I pointed out that I had taken the afternoon off work to see him and I wanted to know why I had been committed. "You were very ill", he said which told me nothing and I kept no more appointments with him. I scoured the library for books on paranoia, schizophrenia and precognitive dreams. If ever there was a subject of the obvious couched in terms of the obscure it was psychiatry. I could not believe that the ill-formed ideas of Sigmund Freud caught popularity in the West and I shared the opinion of those doctors who challenged him. I wonder how he would have fared in ancient Egypt interpreting the Pharaoh's dream with the seven fat cows and seven thin ones, the seven fat ears of corn and the seven thin ones. Egypt would surely have starved with Freud around to propound on the Pharaoh's sex life and those immortal words, "corn in Egypt" never penned to papyrus. William Shakespeare knew more about human behaviour than Freud and his followers and it was not until years later that I obtained a book on CIA experiments with the paranormal did I encounter any publication on the subject to which I could relate. Even then I was stunned that ESP (extra sensory perception) could be controlled so the watcher could go to a given place, my experiences were always random. Interpretation of what was seen was a difficulty, the sightings fragmentary. Dr Chandra Ghosh, with whom I had a rare discussion on the subject, told me that the Russians had spent millions on the subject but achieved nothing.

I was feeling very ill with heavy periods. The GP gave me hormone pills which initially proved a boost and I was optimistic I was better, but later had no effect.

"You'll feel better when your divorce comes through"
the doctor said and I assumed this ailment was
psychosomatic. I was determined to recover so
booked a skiing holiday which I first cancelled after
experiencing a dream that I would break my leg on a
mountain but, after reading an item in *The Sunday
Times* by Professor Eysenck that people who saw into
the future made it happen, reinstated with the
determination to get this nonsense out of my mind.   I
went to Courcheval and broke my ankle coasting to a
halt on an excursion to the next village. "Get up", said
the instructor, "you've not hurt yourself".   I knew my
ankle was broken, I felt it go but was too proud to be
carried back on the blood wagon and did not wish to
hold up the rest of the party. "Go on", I said, "I'll get
myself down". My mind was racing that I had not
beaten the dream premonition but as I had foretold
correctly my brain worked properly.   Surprised the
young man gathered the party together and they skied
off. I was two and a half miles up a mountain, not a
good skier on two legs let alone only one and I was a
bit dazed when I reached the valley where I caught
sight of my reflection in the ski club windows so I took
myself to the hairdressers in the belief that I would be
laid up for a while. At the hairdressers I could feel my
ankle swell; I kept loosening the laces. After I looked
presentable I called a taxi and had the driver take me
back to the chalet to collect my passport and money. I
was in France where I was certain I would not be
treated unless I could show proof of payment. In fact I
was rather more jaundiced than need be and the
driver took me to Docteur Verte who, in his opinion,
was better than the 'opital.   "Where have you been?"
said the doctor who spoke good English and didn't bat
an eyelid when I told him "the hairdressers". I was
feeling really brave by this time and insisted he set it

without an anaesthetic but I must have wriggled, as there was a phone message the next morning to say the X-rays weren't good, I should have no breakfast. The face of the ski instructed when I appeared at the Ski Club with my leg in plaster was a picture. It is forbidden to leave a client in difficulties. I magnanimously exonerated him and took full responsibility but I hope he learnt a lesson not to imagine that all blonds who fall over in the snow do so in the hope of being picked up in his arms. Conceited boy. What I had difficulty understanding was why my leg had broken so easily. It took another thirty years before I realized that excessive haemorrhaging had made my bones brittle. I had osteoporosis.

When the plaster came off, and I got over the horror of seeing a wizened leg, I was referred to the physiotherapy department. Sitting next to me was a lady who had broken her leg on the same mountain; hers too had been set by Docteur Verte. We both commented on his receptionist's ability to act as nurse and anaesthetist and the strangely tough plaster of Paris with blue flecks used to encase our broken limbs. Her husband worked as Administrator at the Royal Free and there was a problem with an Iranian female anaesthetist who didn't like living in the hospital and wanted to live outside with a family to learn English. "I'm not exactly a family", I said, "but I am English and I do have a room to spare if she would like to see it". This is how I met Shookoo, not her real name but, as she said, at the age of twenty-eight she was too old to be called Little Apple Blossom. She moved in and it became apparent very quickly that the reason for the move was not only to learn English (operations at the Royal Free were being conducted in French until her English improved) but also to accommodate her rather large number of boy friends. It was not long before I said something. I picked my words carefully so she could understand the meaning with her limited vocabulary. "Shookoo", I said, "place like bloody brothel".

Her reply was immediate. In broken English she said, "As doctor I understand need for man to keep my 'ormones alive".

I became more shaky and found handing round the teacups to my boss's visitors a nightmare. I solved the problem by letting the gentlemen help themselves from the tray I held with both hands. Dr Stoll insisted my divorce would solve my physical problems; in the meantime I worked, ate, went home to bed and slept as best I could.

One evening I was standing on Bank Station when I heard a voice say, "Sell your shares". The voice was inside my head. I had only a few shares, had little understanding of them but I did understand that the Stock Market fell a few days later and I lost a large proportion of my savings. That shook me. How could I know the Stock Market would fall? Library books said little more than "schizophrenic symptoms indicating conflict in the subconscious", accurate premonitions didn't get a mention. I could accept Prof. Eysenck's pronouncement that I had broken my leg on purpose but doubted I had control of the financial institutions. The Professor was later attacked whilst giving a lecture, the assailant protesting at his opinions on intelligence. Clearly the Professor had not devoted sufficient thought to the outcome of his views, which he expected his minions to accept without reservation.

217

I was certainly ill. I decided I had to leave my job, I really could not cope but before I had worked out the notice my neck swelled up and I collapsed on the Assistant GP's surgery floor. He wondered if I had glandular fever and took a blood test. I got myself home and that night a voice in my head shouted, "Get up. Take some aspirins. Drink plenty of water. Quick". The urgency reached me through the blinding pain and I did as I was told. I also called the doctor. A locum called. He seemed startled when I told him I was making myself ill. My temperature was 103°.

"You *are* ill," he said, "it's not your mind". After the weekend when I rang the GP he sounded concerned. The blood test showed I did not have glandular fever but was severely anaemic. My blood count was a third below what it should be.

It probably sounds strange that I had a doctor as a lodger who had not noticed how ill I was but in truth she was very involved with her own affairs. On the advice of the Americans who wanted to combat the spread of Communism, Daddy had had his palace in Shiraz confiscated by the Shah and the land distributed "to the peasants". Daddy had turned Communist; the exercise was intended to stop the peasants following suit and he was currently in prison and his passport confiscated. To me this was how Communism worked, thus the American advice was counterproductive. Her sister had come over from Switzerland to stay and then her Mother. The mother delighted in answering my telephone although unable to speak English. My friends referred to my Persian invasion. The flow of male friends continued but had reached an impasse the weekend I collapsed when the hospital's varicose vein consultant had invited Shookoo home to dinner and proposed marriage just as one of his female students had turned up screaming hysterically at the door; the consultant had retired temporarily to a monastery to collect his thoughts. My flat became the centre for as many of the consultants' promised brides as Shookoo could uncover, three of them wailed the details of the consultant's proposals. I was treated to lamentations over the colour of her skin; she came from the south and was dark, therefore the Queen Mother had not included her in the marriage list for her son the Shah. Shookoo's school friend Farah Dibah from the north had a fair skin and the Shah had married her. She had gone back home for a holiday to find that two men had asked her family for her hand in marriage without even meeting her. They expected a virgin; she refused to be stitched up for forty pounds. A representative from the Iranian Embassy telephoned her at regular intervals to enquire when she intended returning home to Iran as her country needed her. I wondered what the response would be if our embassy in Washington contacted our doctors working in America and chanted that the DHS needed them. She said that Mr Hawkins my proposed gynaecologist was good. She had worked for him and knew, "He's neat", she said.

The staff at the Royal Free were really nice; gynae wards are prone to be emotional places and the German staff nurse acting, as Sister was a revelation in calming sobbing patients. In all my subsequent brushes with mental health services, I never met any member of staff with such ability. The consultant and registrar restored my shattered faith in the medical profession but I was surprised when they told me to change my GP. "Why?" I said. I knew Henry Stoll had made a mistake but I was better now. I had what is termed a Myectomy, the fibroid was 5cms long and it had come out in one piece so I had not needed a hysterectomy.

"Change your GP", they reiterated.

Shookoo went down with glandular fever and was in another hospital of the Royal Free. Her varicose vein gentleman friend commuted between us carrying messages of good will. Long after she went home and sent me a card to say she had married a doctor and "he quite nice and kind" I had a startling dream. In it Shookoo wore her black Balenciaga coat and was greeting me at Tehran airport. She had asked me to bring medicines but when the boxes draped with the Iranian flag were opened they contained guns. "Zis Janette", she said waving her arms, "is the alternative to ze pill". Three weeks later there was an enormous earthquake in Iran and 20,000 people were killed.

It was while I was staying at Aunt Ena's in Staffordshire that I dreamt my living room ceiling was leaking. The next day I phoned my downstairs neighbour with whom I had left a key and asked her to check if the gas was on. She reported that all was well but three weeks after I returned I came back from work to find water dripping onto the carpet about a foot from the point the leak had been in my dream. It seemed that upstairs had had central heating installed. I never reached a conclusion for the reason for these futuristic dreams but, however terrible the news they foretold, I had comfort in believing that my brain functioned correctly despite professional views to the contrary. Psychiatrists had done an appalling amount of harm with their opinions.

It took a while for me to realize that my extreme lassitude and deep depression was not entirely because of my marital mess. It took six weeks from the operation to be able to sleep without chloral hydrate from which I had difficulty weaning myself. Now I was well I could look after my daughter. My solicitor told me I required affidavits from my doctors ascertaining I was well. Well. Henry Stoll's was not possible to process, he didn't even sign it and seemed to muddle reference to my mother with me, "extreme concern about her daughter" did not relate to my concern for my daughter – but charged five guineas – and McNeil – for even more guineas – provided two statements. One said I was unfit to have care of my daughter and the second, intimating that he had panicked at the news how anaemic I became, that I had a normal blood count when admitted for his treatment. "Change your doctor", said my solicitor.

I had a dream that Dr Henry Stoll was waiting for me. I went to see him. He was wearing the same suit and tie that he had worn in my dream. He had sitting by him a female Jewish assistant and he batted off, "I am so sorry for you, you have been so ill". For some reason, tears welled up and I started to cry. He went on that there wasn't anything really wrong with me but he didn't want to be involved in marital disputes. He didn't think he'd hear from me again after he sent me the statement. "I hope you get custody of your child, your husband's totally unsuitable". He thus disclosed that he had met my husband although he was not John's doctor. He confirmed what I had suspected, the eye doctor had panicked, applied to Henry Stoll with a garbled story and Stoll, perhaps in good faith, had interviewed John in such a way as to topple him over mentally which caused a diversion from the main issue. As I closed the surgery door, through my tears, I could see Stoll was laughing. I had to restrain myself not to rush back in and grab him.   From thereon I campaigned to have an enquiry into my committal to Horton.   Not least of my complaint was that I had been treated for mental illness for two years when I had severe gynaecological problems.   It was some time before I learned that Stoll had been reprimanded by the surgical team at the Royal Free for delayed referral to them and was smarting from it.

I had had the same GP, Dr Ramsey, who brought me into the world for twenty-four years until I married. London doctors seemed very different to those practicing in rural areas. Henry Stoll was my second GP since moving to NW3, I had discovered the first operated what could be termed a very low-key surgery and kept no records.   Henry Stoll at least had an efficient set-up. The next one I approached asked for my history. When I mentioned the eye doctor he leapt from his desk and cowered against the wall shouting, "I can't have you as a patient. I have a wife and children to think of". He did accept me on condition I saw his social worker, who was a kind woman but preferred no help whatever in helping me solve the mystery of my committal. I had been prepared to forgive and forget, everybody makes mistakes, but I could not condone the attitude and behaviour of the medical profession to cover their errors.   At work an employee had taken a phone call to renew a policy and gone home and forgotten it. There was a large claim and the policy was non-existent.   The company could have denied taking the original phone call but it had integrity and much of its business was derived from its reputation.   They paid up, the sum costly. The employee was not fired but an overhaul of the renewal process was instigated so that the error did not reoccur. Why did the medical profession take so much time covering up their errors instead of straightening them out?

My solicitor begged me not to sue. "We have some terrible cases", he said, "The medical profession are ghastly. They hold hands." The replies I received from those in authority were just evasive words, "You have complained outside the statutory time limit of six weeks" from Family Practitioners (I had complained immediately I understood the situation).
"We look to other authorities such as DHS to deal with your complaint" from the General Medical Council (GMC). "Doctors are responsible for their own clinical treatment" from the Department of Health who took at least eight weeks to respond at all. "We are satisfied that the correct procedure regarding your committal was adhered to" from the Area Health Authority. I phoned the GMC and spoke to the Secretary. I understood that I was expected to be flattered their letter had been signed by the President. "You can't sue them can you?" I said. The Secretary agreed. "The only thing that's left is to take the law into one's own hands," I said. "That's right," said the Secretary.

I took a while to pluck up courage to do it. I broke a milk bottle but it was too jagged and could do serious damage. I broke another one and clutching the neck end of the remains I stood outside Henry Stoll's surgery waiting for him to come out. I was amazed when he smiled and stepped forward to greet me. He didn't smile for long. I hit him. He backed away and I advanced menacingly brandishing the remains of the bottle. I then went home and waited for the police to call and arrest me. If I couldn't sue the medical profession I would at least get them to court to do some explaining. After a couple of days I presented myself at the Police Station and told the man behind the desk what I had done. He looked at me rather oddly and went away to make a telephone call. When he came back he said, "Dr Stoll's gone away for a few days to recover and get the glass out of his head. Now look. You've had a hard time. You're to go home and forget about it". I was most upset. What I had gone through to pluck up courage to do what I did was something I could not face again. Stoll wasn't going to get away with ruining my life by saying he forgave me, not when I had seen him laughing. What a cop out. What could I do? I had to do something. I went home and wrote a letter to McNeil at Horton I told him what I had done to Henry Stoll and asked again for the reason why I had been committed.

A few days later the police called and I was under arrest. At the Magistrate's Court I said my daughter was coming for the weekend and I had promised to take her to the Lord Mayor's Show and it would be a big disappointment if I wasn't available. I got bail and we had a lovely weekend.

On Monday I was dismayed when James Baird, the social worker arrived, the one born in a mental hospital who had taken me to Horton. He marched into my flat, demanded I make him a cup of coffee; I was not reassured with this but seemed to have no other options, "Now listen. We'll play this low key. You don't want the press involved and then we'll sort it out much more quickly. Leave it to me". I had no idea what he was talking about or intended to do but if this meant that I would receive an explanation for the destruction in my life then I would co-operate. I didn't exactly co-operate, I was more swung along with his enthusiasm. A lawyer was laid on, a doctor called in and this time it was to Friern Barnet that I was sent. The episode taught me never, ever, trust the glib assurances of a psychiatric social worker but even on the way there he was telling me, "Hospitals sort these things out much quicker than the courts". Perhaps he believed what he was saying. I remember a fellow at the tennis club who really believed he had been in a Japanese POW camp, had bombed Berlin and fought in North Africa. The truth was he had served the entire war in Bushey Fire Brigade. As we entered the ward James Baird called out to the Charge Nurse, "This is a good one. I'll tell you all about it".

Apart from being the longest building in England, a mile long, Friern was different to Horton. It was a mixed ward and a small allowance by DHS to each patient made the begging for cigarettes a thing of the past. The patients were mainly reasonably dressed, lolled around in armchairs all day and cadged cigarettes off their fellows more from boredom than necessity or desperation.

One man's wife had died. He needed a home help for his children but the social worker, James Baird, had had him committed. At medicine times he would say, "More Smarties", and then sleep till the next mealtime. He was lucky his teenage sons had been well brought up; they visited Dad regularly and clearly wanted him back home. .

I was given drugs – Stelazine again, which made my hands shake. I went along with the routine. There was an American ex-serviceman on the ward, a Korean veteran who had flown thirty-two missions over Germany in World War II as a rear gunner in Flying Fortresses. We owed our lives to men like him. He had been in a car crash with somebody on the base and his wife thought he should receive compensation; to this end he sought the help of the camp psychiatrist since when he had been discharged from the Army Air Force and been in thirty-two mental hospitals both here and in the States. Telling me about it he said, "I was sent to a mental hospital a thousand miles from base and my family. I played cards twenty three hours a day". With his severance pay he had bought a tobacconists off an ex man friend of Aunty Joyce, in Bushey High Street, not popular with his wife who didn't smoke. In all the years of living in London I had only met three people who had ever heard of Bushey, one was a fellow in a City insurance office, the second a guide in Istanbul who had lived in Bushey for six months to learn English and now a third who was American. He was keen on golf so a crowd of us went to a practice site and hit golf balls off a platform and in the evenings visited the pub. Most of the day we sat around playing cards or scrabble. After a few weeks I was allowed home for the weekends and I would invite half a dozen or so of the ward for lunch. They would call in at a local pub and arrive to eat after closing time. One of the gang was a young accountant, a brilliant mathematician, who had woken up from a park bench not knowing where or who he was. His memory had returned after a couple of weeks and it was patently a terrible shock to him to realise he had fourteen days for which he could not account but, as the psychiatrists had no explanation for the event and could do nothing for him it did seem sad that he was being kept in wasting his life away.

My section was for a year and a day but three consultants, three registrars and three months later I was pronounced fit to leave. I gazed in wonderment at the latest registrar, an Egyptian called Macar. My hands shook so much I could not hold a cup to my mouth, I have to lean down to drink. "I have still had no explanation for being committed to Horton". A flicker of apprehension crossed the man's face. "You are a lady", he said, "You go away and live your life". "With a mental stigma?" I said. He closed the file and smiled.

James Baird organised me a GP who said she would not take me as a patient unless I took my psychiatric medication. I drew the prescriptions to keep her happy and dumped them in the waste bin. Three months later I was back in a gynae ward having yet another op, a minor scrape this time having run away in terror at a consultant gynaecologist at University Hospital who, after looking at my file and saying "You've been to Horton" added, "you should have it all out. You can't want it for anything". I gazed upwards at him, it was an effort not to tell the man that I doubted his was much use either and why didn't he have the lot off. The GP to whom I retold the story referred me to a female consultant and all was well. Stelazine did seem to upset my hormones and the medical profession did seem to gloss over the matter. I tried to pick up the threads but I was bothered not just by the committal to Horton but by the ease errors of clinical judgement are evaded. The courts seemed to accept the cover-ups. I tried to live normally which was difficult with the wall I built to protect myself from people knowing where I had been. If I had been honest about the mental committals I would not have been able to get employment. I felt sick when I had the local rates bill. Friern Barnet cost £6M in 1972. I approved of refuse emptying, libraries, drainage, police and so on but not social workers and mental hospitals. I deducted 13p:£ which was my contribution to social services.

Scientology had been in the news because it had been labelled a harmful organisation by psychiatrists. Any enemy of psychiatry, I thought, is a friend of mine and so I contacted them. I found them helpful and sympathetic and at no time did they push me to join their Church. They were compiling a dossier on psychiatric case histories and I let them have mine. Their information included a story of a husband and wife whose GP told them their local psychiatrist had appealed to him for "more intelligent patients". They had great difficulty extricating themselves from the psychiatrist.

The *Sunday Times* had an item about Mental Patients' Union and I went to see them. They were ensconced in a squat house in Mayola Road, Hackney, the set up run by a communist sociologist and his Maoist wife. A poster of Stalin dominated one room. The road was designated for redevelopment and the life of the house was in the lap of advancing bulldozers. Police were regular visitors sometimes for disturbances caused by desperate absconding patients and other times for purposes of routine surveillance. The leader was well versed in relative aspects of the law. I was considered odd as I had a "respectable" flat, slept in my own bed, not a mattress on the floor and had a job. They had limited funds but had meetings, gave floor space and meals to the desperate; all I met there had stories to tell of psychiatric treatment, the leader attributing the situation to a capitalist society. I was not so sure. There was psychiatry in Russia. I could not believe that I had been incarcerated and my health wrecked for drug manufacturers' profit. Most of the people in the squat house saw a psychiatrist regularly to ensure sickness chits for Social Security benefits, some vowed never to work in a capitalist society. In vain I protested that it was mutts like me, not wicked capitalists, who were paying taxes for their benefits. It was at one of their smoke-filled meetings that I felt something more tangible had to be done than rant about mental hospital horrors.

I set up a petition for the Abolition of Forced Psychiatric Treatment made up of forty two statements showing that people were worse off after treatment than they were before, the best that could be said was that it made no difference at all. I was disappointed I could not collect more but was later assured that the response had been remarkably good for psychiatric patients; several refused to participate as they feared repercussions and reprisals. One man had undergone psychoanalysis during which he murdered his father; another member of his family had been to the same analyst and hung himself; the analyst had gone to New Zealand.   Another man had been in the Merchant Navy; off S .America he had had a voice in the head which he thought was the Chief Engineer maligning him; he had burst into the Chief's cabin and berated him and was put off the ship at Vancouver, flown home, put in a mental hospital and given ECT without anaesthetic. He had lost his ticket so could no longer work on ships and ended up walking from Scotland to London living off dustbins and doing occasional prison terms for loitering and breaking and entering.   Several people thought the petition would be a breakthrough, "You're the first one to do something", Bill Warwick had written. He was really hopeful that his shocking experiences would be recognised. He also campaigned on behalf of his sister's husband given LSD with disastrous results. DHS had written, "The results of this treatment are disappointing". When I phoned the police about delivering the petition to Harold Wilson at No.10 the voice the other end said, "You need to be a foreigner to get anything done in this Town".

I had attended a meeting at which Viktor Fineberg, a Russian dissident arrested for protesting at the Russian invasion of Czechoslovakia, had spoken of his experiences in a Russian mental hospital. With a population of over two hundred and thirty million, Russia had nineteen such institutions, "Ireland's got twenty two", whispered my friend.
 The UK had well over a hundred. Viktor Fineberg had escaped with his female psychiatrist – he had a stronger stomach than me. He held up a list of British psychiatrists who had petitioned the Russian Government for his release. The audience applauded when I said, "It's pot calling the kettle black". When the tumult died down I explained to Fineberg, "It means they are the same" and he smiled his understanding. "It doesn't matter what corner of the world we come from", I continued, "it's a certain type of person who is pilloried for standing up to what is evil" and the applause broke out again. Later he was joined in this country by Bukovsky who renounced psychiatry very strongly but ended up living with the practitioner who had accompanied Fineberg out.

I was taken to a spiritualist meeting in Kentish Town. The medium was a man called Benjamin who certainly provoked discussion. If he was a fraud he was a good one. He had recently recovered from a heart attack reminding the congregation that he had not been able to divulge his occupation on the hospital admission forms. The audience murmured their understanding. His eyes strayed round the hall and, directing his attention to about the middle of the second row he said, "I smell sawdust. Does this mean anything to you?". A woman in his line of vision spoke up, "My father was a carpenter". The message from Dad sounded trivial but the woman was happy with it. He then focused in my direction and said to a fellow sitting next to me, "I've a message from your mother" the young man confirmed that his mother was dead, "She says don't worry about your father he's all right. What happened? You put him in a care home?"

"Yes" said the youth, "I couldn't cope with him".

"Well she says don't upset yourself about that but she's worried you've too many girl friends. You should settle down with one". The young man accepted the message in silence.

Benjamin eyes roamed round the hall narrowly identifying the road in which a person lived – "You live on the Finchley Road" he would say to be told, "I live in a turning off it". He told one woman she had just had a vision and she confirmed that she had, the vision of Benjamin's mother telling him not to overdo it. The friend who took me to the meeting had received a message on a previous occasion. She had been told that she had reached the end of a long dark tunnel. "To start at the beginning of another one?" she laughed to me. We both agreed it was difficult to invent such near accurate messages for such a large gathering and keep going for a good hour. I decided to take along Tony from Mayola Road who had experienced voices on board ship. "This man", I told him, "has all the schizophrenic symptoms, he has voices, visions, imaginary smells but he's rational and sane". I was disappointed when Tony fell asleep soon after we arrived at the meeting and just jolted back to consciousness near the end. On the way out he said, "I never thought the dead would send such trivial messages".

My mother was a problem. My father had died and although upset she had seemed happy enough going away to hotels for breaks with her birthday sister, my Aunty Ena who was also widowed. I had a call from Aunty E who had dreamt my mother was in trouble and next day had gone to untold lengths to obtain the telephone number of a next-door neighbour who told her my mother was in Exminster mental hospital. It seemed that a social worker had been laid on after my father died and not taken kindly to having the door slammed in her face with the words, "Not today thank you" and continued to call. She had broken into my mother's apartment overlooking the River Exe to find my mother in a heap on the floor. Callously I would have left her there to sober up; she would not have allowed herself to get into that state twice. The social worker had had my mother committed and searched through the flat for evidence of alcohol and had discovered a wrapped empty gin bottle in the dustbin. My parents always wrapped their rubbish. If the social worker had discovered a full bottle I would think the situation warranted a committal. My mother came to in a mental hospital, which must have been a horrible shock. She called the grinning man wearing a white coat the steward and psychiatrist the butler. She had never appreciated slapstick humour, hers was always of the verbal kind. The psychiatrist was not amused; he was used to dealing with widowed old ladies.

He contacted the Official Solicitor to have her "estate" taken over to ensure payment to an old people's home. I trailed down to Devonshire, I trailed back again. Unannounced I visited the Court of Protection to be told that I was the first person ever to visit these offices and that, unless I had a legal or medical qualification, there was nothing either my mother or I could do. The judge altered the date of the hearing, did not notify me of the new date and another *fait accompli* sealed my mother's destiny. All because I had been committed to Horton. I was really angry but also frightened. There seemed to be a power in the land that was driving me and mine downwards.

The banging was so uncouth I almost didn't open it but when I did I was pushed over as two men barged in. "Who are you?" I cried from a position on the floor.

"The Police" replied the larger of the two men, "can I use the phone?" he added. I understood that he would use it whether I said he could or not. He called in a psychiatrist, another doctor, social worker and, five hours later, a female policewoman. "I had two break-ins in a week and this block of four flats had had four in six weeks", I said. "It's amazing that you people don't catch anybody but can spend all this time here when I've done nothing at all". This social worker was called Heevy who sat on my pale blue velvet-nursing chair with his legs splayed out in a really ugly posture. "What's happened to James Baird?" I enquired.

"He's died". I was surprised. "Natural causes", he added hastily. He accompanied me to Friern. "Broadmoor" he leered. He did not elucidate what he meant.

This time Friern Barnet was different. A locked mixed ward, the male dormitory constructed from the corridor through which everybody had to walk to reach the office. I gasped as my first impression was a row of black eyes and plastered limbs it was like a casualty department. I was terrified that these accidents had happened inside the institution. The television blared deafeningly. I was taken to see the Registrar, Dr Perchaud. "Why am I here?" I enquired.

"The police haven't told us", he replied.

"Why don't you ask them?"

"Oh they never tell us". If this was true how could he treat anybody. The question of medication arose. "You don't have to take it but I must put something on your card" he reassured. His assurance was short-lived. At a subsequent medicine round the Charge Nurse said I must take my medicine. I refused and he threatened to have me injected. Much to my amazement the tougher male patients, prison transfers, moved closer silently and the Charge Nurse backed off. He did not mention the subject again.

At the best of times people can be difficult but when they are cooped up in those conditions they are intolerable. Windows which opened only a few inches were smashed, the TV set went flying, the record player survived temporarily. One fellow caught stealing a motorbike to get home after a party was prescribed Stelazine; he said he'd stay until he got his teeth. Another was singing for his supper on a bus; he was prescribed Largactil. One man had smashed his car when drunk and was still suffering from the trauma and said little. I discovered that all the plaster casts and black eyes on the ward had been caused by accidents sustained outside. One night there was a fire. Being in a locked ward on the top floor with somebody lighting a bonfire beneath their bed in the dormitory is good practice for the nerves

Once a week the clinical ward round of approximately ten staff was held in the female dormitory; one week it was very draughty as two windows had been broken and it was a cool November. I attended one of these meetings at which I learned nothing. No reason for the committal or date for release was given.

I had received a couple of telephone messages from well-wishers, particularly those at Mayola Road and my downstairs neighbour came to visit me. She was clearly appalled at the situation I was in but confirmed that the social worker James Baird had indeed died of cancer, "He went quite mad and his wife left him before he passed away". A nurse told me somebody had phoned and would I ring them back, the patients' call box was downstairs by the main entrance. The nurse who escorted me wandered off and I took the opportunity to escape. I walked five miles to friends where I was advised I should stay hidden for a month, until the section expired. The friends tried to find out why I'd been sectioned but got nowhere. The Police Superintendent had by this time been moved to another Station, the third in as many months but when tracked down said, "The police need somewhere to live", which was mystifying. I came to the conclusion that it was a combination of suppressing the reason for my rates non-payment and the petition to No.10 plus my name had apparently been on the police station list from the Stoll incident and the police needed to show they had arrest figures to qualify their existence. If the block of flats I lived in was a guide, every household in Hampstead experienced a burglary every twenty four weeks.

Once the committal section was void I visited with a friend to collect my belongings to find most of them, including my money, had been stolen. I then went down to Devonshire to see my mother in her old people's home. I stayed in her flat and the Official Solicitor wrote and demanded rent from me. In all the years until she died my Mother never once sent me or her only grandchild a birthday or Christmas present. Her funds were certainly well guarded to pay her fees.

I went to see her by two buses that ran twice a week and it took nearly two hours to travel the crow-flying twelve miles. The nursing home was in a pleasant spot but remote and overcrowded. My mother was missing her fur coat, diamond ring and watch. She didn't actually ask for them but kept looking at her vacant wrist for the time and looking at her ringless hands. The social worker said she would look into the matters – the coat never turned up but the other items materialised in safe keeping at Exminster Hospital. I arranged for her to be brought to Topsham to her flat for lunch where I sadly realised I could not cope with her for a longer period. She was totally distrait and suffering from shock. Reluctantly I told her I was going for McNeil. "Good luck", she said, "I didn't live through two world wars to be treated like this" So we parted amicably. That was the last time we met.

The night before I went back to London I had a nightmare. I read the details in the taxi driver's paper as he took me to the station. I dreamt the IRA had attacked the Ideal Home Exhibition. I'd had an ideal home. I dreamt something else but it was a long time before I realised that I had foreseen the advent of

AIDS. Why should I dream this? What good does it do when I could do nothing about the things I foresaw.

I bought a vegetable knife and took a train to Epsom. It was as though the fates did not want me to go. The train had been wrongly sign-posted and I had to change trains to reach my destination. I walked stoically through the alley way en route to Horton and stationed myself along the corridor about lunch time. I thought a vegetable knife was symbolic for McNeil who treated me like a cabbage. I had been to see him a couple of years previously by appointment in a last ditch attempt to get him to talk. He had had with him a young Irish registrar to whom he tried showing off by displaying disdain for my request. He recited to me his notes where I had said that the reason for the committal was to provide him with patients. I recalled how Henry Stoll had reduced me to tears. I sat back in the chair, relaxed, "You look much better", I said sweetly, "That twitch of yours is much improved". Practically immediately one side of his face contorted uncontrollably. He was clearly thrown. "You. You..." he stuttered waving his fist at me as his face contorted again. The Irish Registrar looked amused at him and I had got out as quickly as I could.

He hadn't changed. As he passed me in the corridor I poked him in the backside and was surprised when he continued walking without a shudder. It was like poking a sausage. Perhaps the knife had not gone in. Had I imagined stabbing him. He turned, glared and shook a finger at me, "Now don't do that again", he said.

I had intended to poke him once only but I could imagine him telling people how he had staved off the attack single handed with a wagging finger. I poked him again and a fight ensued. For a split second I thought he was inviting me to kill him, which I had no intention of so doing. I wanted him alive and understanding the damage he had caused. He tottered back to his office clutching himself squeaking, "Call an ambulance. Call an ambulance". I stood in the doorway and when he saw me he looked absolutely terrified.

"It's all right", I said, "I'm not going to stab you again". I gave the knife to a receptionist and a grinning nurse asked, "Why did you do it".

"Because he ruined my life and drove my mother to drink". Nobody seemed particularly shocked, just incredulous and grinning. I wanted to get McNeil to court and this was the only way I could do it. It took me a long while to realise the significance of his remaining standing. He was not collapsed in a heap on the floor. He was standing up unaided.

The police came and took me away in a Panda car with an Alsatian sitting in the back. They were kind and seemed to comprehend what I had endured and was attempting to do. They took me to the local cottage hospital to have my thumb stitched; as it was being done a psychiatrist walked in. "Go away. Go away", I said but he just stood gazing above my head with a stupid smirk like he'd won a battle. At a time like this why couldn't I have protection from these stupid people who thought they could rule the world.

The Magistrate's hearing was next day. I had not slept well. Before we went I was handed a charge sheet. I was shaken when I read "Attempted Murder". The bacon sandwich I was given seemed rather salty and the coffee tasted odd but it might have been the state I was in that was affecting my taste buds. I started to feel ill when we reached court, my movements were strangely jerky and I realised I was incontinent. I did my best to rectify the problems and tried to appear relaxed when appearing in court where the hearing was merely a formality. The three magistrates looked ill, tense and pale. They gave the impression of being in a state of shock. After a long wait in the graffiti covered cells – how few who had been there liked the police - I was put in a Black Maria; I thought I was going to be sick on the journey, I felt really ill by the time we arrived at Holloway Prison. The Reception Nurse looked at me and said, "Is your face always that colour?". There was no mirror available but I gathered I looked yellow but flushed. The little Iranian doctor flicked through some papers and suddenly burst into tears. Sympathy for what I had endured maybe. "Dr Perchaud", she gasped through her sobs, "'e is a very nice man".

Dr. Perchaud was the Registrar at Friern where I had been taken by the Police after delivering the petition to No.10. He was a personable young man, "I'm sure he is", I murmured through the nausea, "I'm sure he's charming socially. I only know him as a patient". Her tears prevented her seeing that I was in need of medical attention; when I was taken to a cell it was after lock-up. When the door clanged behind me I just flopped onto the bed, I felt dreadful. I blacked out and came to and blacked out again. There was a burst of light, my spirit floated across the cell leaving my lifeless body on the bed. During the flash as I died I heard the voice of the policeman at Epsom Station telling me that it was they who had poisoned me. In a flash of clarity I knew that the police had been provided with the drug by another source. In my suspended state I knew I could float through the solid wall but my brain told me, "I've got to stay alive. I've got to tell people what's happening. What would they pin on me if I were dead?". So I stopped floating and came back; as I re-entered my body all went black.

I came to, struggled up and rang the call button, which made a tag flop down, by my cell. The snag was that many of the girls weren't sleepy when they were banged up and amused themselves pressing their call buttons to the extent that most calls were ignored. A nurse eventually approached. I explained I'd blacked out. Rules prevented her entering the cell alone, there was a low ratio of night staff but she fetched me a beaker of water. I took a sip and collapsed on the floor. I came to, soaked, the water spilt. Sheer willpower got me up from the floor and onto the bed. After a while a voice from the door enquired if I was all right. "I think so", I said and drifted into sleep.

The next day I could hardly stand up, my hands and feet were blue but I did manage to get into the main room for breakfast. I noticed the metal walls were stamped HMP Hull, it gave inkling that those in authority felt even the walls could be nicked and were required to be labelled. Hull? I staggered back to my cell and a nurse called a psychiatrist, Dr Colin Sherry; as he entered my cell a prisoner called out, "He's f.... useless". The doctor glanced at my feet and hands and said, "Tell me, do you write poetry". The nurse was clearly appalled and fetched another doctor, this time sari-dressed who refused to even enter the cell. "Drink plenty of water and flush whatever it is out of your system" she said as she stood by the grill. This was the best and only medical advice I received in Holloway Prison despite seeing twelve different doctors over twenty times, it being obligatory to be given the once over going out and coming back from appearances in court. For a while my head felt stuffed with cotton wool, I had no sensation of thinking, moving, I spoke and heard my voice and that's how I knew I was talking. The sensations were most strange. I found I came up in a rash even after eating a boiled egg and came to the conclusion that every organ in my body had been affected by the drugging.

I was in the same cell occupied by Ruth Ellis before she was hanged and the ward sister was the same now as then. Zara, my downstairs neighbour came to see me, "The last time I came here", she said woefully, "was to see dear Ruth" who had shot her lover George Blakely outside our local pub, the Magdala on Parliament Hill. "they wouldn't let me leave you a bottle of wine" she commiserated.

Suddenly I was removed from the main admittance ward and put in the Obs; I gathered I was now under a Section 43, no contact with other prisoners, lock-up was at 4 p.m. instead of the usual 7.30, the lavatories filthy beyond belief and exercise in the fresh air and sunshine now minimal instead of frequent. Why those destined for Broadmoor were treated in this inhuman segregated manner was never explained and at the time I did not know that was where I was destined to go. Even visits were no longer in the Portakabin but on the ward with a wardress either side of the table, any privacy was accidental. The friends who came to see me had a tale to tell when they left – at least one was clearly mystified and terrified - and could have no doubt that I was being singled out. I was later joined in my isolation by a young girl in for infanticide who in years to come would co-habit with the consultant psychiatrist who would accept her into his care. Meanwhile she was disturbed she was heading for Broadmoor. It was a hot summer, the windows had nearly all been broken to provide fresh air and most of my neighbours were what could be described as juvenile sub-normals. One of these came up to my door and asked why I was there.

"Because I'm dangerous", I said and to prove it barked "woof woof" through the bars.

"I'm more dangerous than you", she said and proved it, the proof lasting for the next forty eight hours. At the end of that time there wasn't a Bible in the place that hadn't had all its pages torn out and the whole block was swimming in bits of torn paper and urine. I was amazed when the senior doctor, a Greek gynaecologist, arrived to view the disturbance with Dr Sherry. They both seemed happy at the mess and were clearly enjoying the spectacle of juveniles subjugating themselves through reasons of boredom.

If a social worker like James Baird could rig a Magistrates Court, then what couldn't a psychiatrist do with a Crown Court. I had learned one important lesson. British justice is best at hiding its injustices, that's why it is the best in the world. The solicitor's clerk, a retired policeman of the kindly old-fashioned type, came to see me bearing chocky bars to soften me up. He showed me the court statements and I nearly had a fit. "I never said I stabbed him again, again and again". "He's in Intensive Care", he said. The statement at Epsom Police Station dwelled mainly on the transport I used to get there. "This is invented and makes me look like a raving lunatic" I protested. He agreed but didn't seem inclined to do anything about it. I decided to change my solicitor. Holloway had changed its Governor. "Don't worry", the new one assured me, "it'll be fine. I've just come from Brixton where there are a thousand men on remand all wanting to change their solicitors". After returning from rare exercise outside a few days later I found that the reports brought in from the solicitors had been switched for others. If before I had sounded like a raving lunatic now I was a Noel Coward sophisticate. Instead of there being a female witness now there was a statement by a man. Dr Henry Stoll still had difficulty discerning the difference between my mother and I. A psychiatrist at Friern said I had been someone else's patient. The number of stabbings had been reduced. What was going on. Did the Director of Criminal Prosecutions employ script writers? Why this farce when I was pleading guilty but wanted the circumstances examined?

The clerk from the solicitors visited again. "I thought you might be interested in these", he said. "These" were an assortment of telegrams, postcard, and bits of paper all, apparently purported to have been sent by me to Henry Stoll and some psychiatrist I'd never met. One rambling telegram referred to Pinky and Perky (a children's TV programme), the postcard in my handwriting with a Weston postmark (I'd never been to Weston) read, "And what kind of contraception do you use?". It took some pondering and working out.

"Why hasn't anybody shown me these before or mentioned them?" I said, "I've asked often enough. Do you mean to tell me that these bits of paper were the reason I was committed to Horton without a trial or explanation to have my life wrecked". It was slowly filtering through, odd events like playing consequences with so-called friends and bottles of wine. My husband, good at art and I had already

243

discovered he had forged my name on an insurance policy, and my mother had been horrified I'd left him but the split would not have occurred without the rape and Henry Stoll interfering and upsetting my ex. I'd not made a mistake and aimed at the wrong cause. My parents' horror at my demands they help me were now understood. Oh dear. What a mess. Those bits of paper were pretty innocuous and not sufficient to commit anybody. They would not stand scrutiny in court. So why I had I been committed without any explanation. No wonder McNeil and those at Friern had dodged the issue and hoped I'd go away. What is mad? If psychiatry had not existed could I have survived. The answer is 'Yes'. All McNeil had had to do was remove the mental stigma and explain the situation to me. Instead his handling, accusing my Mother of being the cause, despite her part in the telegram sending, drove her to drink and made everything worse. An explanation was what I had hoped for but I had not expected anything like this. As far as I was concerned that episode was now closed. What had haunted and molested me had gone away and for ever after I slept at night without night sedation. What remained was to try to stop the concealment of bad medical practices to the detriment of the subject.

Some of the journeys to and from court were nice. One policeman drove the scenic route along the Embankment to show me the newly painted bridges for the Silver Jubilee. He regaled his companion and me with stories of his experiences in the Army based on the Rhine, how he'd lost his way during a storm in the Baltic and hailed a passing German merchant ship to enquire the way to Hamburg. "How did you win the war with navigation that bad" shouted back the

German captain. The policeman and companion asked if they could take me to Epsom again but that was the last time I saw them. One tall wardress stared at me and enquired if she had taken me to court before. She stood for a while then her face cleared and she said, "Janet Coleman", my maiden name, "you used to have fair hair" it had turned brown with age. I stared blankly.

"Don't you recognise me", she said smiling. "Audrey Covey". I knew her name but had not recognised her face.

"The best goalie in the hockey team" I laughed. We both lived in Bushey but different parts of it, my Mother had taught at the school in the road where Audrey lived.

The day of the Old Bailey hearing arrived and I met the barrister, Mr O'Rourke, for the first time. He listened for a while, it was a very hot day, "Do you mind if I take this off", he said removing his wig. "Please do" I said and it set the seal.

The charge of Attempted Murder was quickly substituted for Grievous Bodily Harm; I did not realise at the time that by doing this the court could be assured that I would plead guilty and not have a jury. I did not know that newspaper restrictions had not been removed so there would be no journalist in court. Anyway Stonehouse (ex Postmaster General) was in the next court in his fifty something day, allowed to conduct his own case, the Press would not be interested in my protest. I wanted to plead Mitigating Circumstances but I was told that the Judge would not like this. Only later did I understand that it mattered little what the judge liked. "There's nothing I can do for you", said the barrister, "your crime is against the

Establishment. "What did you think of the psychiatrist I sent in to see you?" he asked casually.

I had refused to have any psychiatric reports submitted on my behalf as I challenged the entire profession, I certainly could not accept having one of them speak up for me. "For a woman of my age to be represented by somebody looking like a white-suited gigolo would not have gone down well in court apart from the fact that I can't stand any of them", I said. The barrister looked amused. "He's my brother-in-law", he said, "he's married to my sister".

The judge looked like a white rabbit and the proceedings began. I was shattered that it seemed he had been briefed to give me life imprisonment, he mentioned it a couple of times. I could not believe that the prosecuting barrister was reading the original statements, the ones that had been left in my cell had been to keep me quiet. The Epsom policeman knew nothing about my being administered any unidentified potion surreptitiously and stepped down from the stand. Dr Colin Sherry stepped up, he stated I was psychotic and referred to a report by a Dr Roper whose report I had not seen whose name I had not learned in Holloway when he interviewed me with the words, "I'm here to write a report for the Home Office to send you to a mental hospital".

Idly the barrister enquired of Dr Sherry, "Why, when Mrs Cresswell's problems emanate from psychiatric treatment do you recommend more?". A simple question.

Dr Sherry reacted violently. He banged the side of the box and shouted, "She needs treatment. She needs treatment". The court went silent. The barrister

246

resembled a puppy straining on a lead as he barked, "To hand up a knife is not psychosis. To stab him at his surgery to avoid upsetting his family at home is not psychosis. You say she can't communicate. I've just had one and a half hours perfectly lucid conversation with her. What's wrong with you? She's a very brave woman to do what she did. She's not mentally ill, she's suffering from diseases in the minds of the medical profession".

The judge woke up and leaned out of his box to say "ECT is very controversial isn't it?" He looked helplessly at the barrister and said, "I've got to send her somewhere". He didn't give me life imprisonment as he had been briefed to do but he did send me to Broadmoor with an indefinite sentence. He did allow me to say a few words at the end of the trial and I took the opportunity to challenge psychiatric definitions. If a person had no degree of paranoia they were foolhardy; schizophrenia, containing an element of seeing into the future could be diagnosed as inventing things by those without the ability of foresight. To be without this gift produced mental myopia. To be condemned as insane by those with mental myopia was insanity, and so on. Mention of "life imprisonment" was omitted from the committal order.

The next day in Holloway the social worker, a Mrs Stearn who had refused the offer to become Governor of Holloway, dropped by. "The doctors are very frightened", she said.

"I can't think why", I replied, "it's me who's going to Broadmoor, not them".

There is a rule whereby prisons must fulfil the court rulings within three weeks so three weeks later I was on my way to Crowthorne. All the ward were locked in their cells as I was led out to the waiting van. A kindly nurse asked if I would mind if she put in for escort as she wanted to see what Broadmoor was like. She had two sons with cerebral palsy and, although she could cope with one child at home, she could not care for two so they were both in care. Her husband had left her saying "A dog has more intelligence than my sons". It was incredibly sad that a fraction of the money it cost to keep two children in care would provide more than ample home assistance.

We got in the van before somebody remembered my valuables had not been collected. A nurse went and fetched them. Then my coat and dress, removed by Epsom Police had been sent by them to the cleaners and these had been forgotten and had to be collected from somewhere else. I hadn't wondered why the Police had sent my clothing to the cleaners but I gasped when confronted with my check coat. It had several yellow marks; could it be that if I had obtained bail I would have been luminous in the dark to be picked up easily when I collapsed in the street on the way home, as I must surely have done. I never discovered what the substance was or why the coat was so marked.

CHAPTER 11 – BROADMOOR

Hope is Eternal

I was unable to thank the reporter for the box of chocolates she left; I was a bit dubious – there was a distinct bloom on them as though she had had them some time.

My friend has brought me in another of those four-portion Waitrose cakes so I take it down later to Alvada and we consume it over the usual coffee served in her large Wedgwood mugs. I hesitate to tell her of the secret recording session in the Central Hall; I dare not tell anybody although by some viewpoints it had been authorized. I wonder how the staff will react when they learn that their entry banning has been ignored and the reporter came in via the psychiatrist. It is hard to find much that is sane in the way the worst patients are got out because nobody can stand them; the more acceptable can stay in the system far longer. It is as though those who make-believe the drugs have cured them – how can a dose of Largactil cure a person with relatives who are physically ill, one with a brain tumour, and murders them to put them out of their misery – stand a chance of getting out. Those honest enough to say the drugs make them drowsy, put on weight, make their hands shake and they still have the same feelings do not stand a chance. The situation is insane.

Alvada is more resigned to her situation than I am, though more bitter, and in my "the grass is always greener on the other side" mood I wonder how much her Civil Service background, even though it's

American and surely more generous and efficient than our own, contributes to acceptance of government red tape and the legislation that keeps us both detained.

The TV film is shown some weeks later entitled *Insane Justice*. Most of the ward, including staff, appeared in the day room to watch it, not a terribly good idea as the chatter and cheering drowned quite a lot of the commentary and it was difficult to pick up the nuances. It opened with shots of the high perimeter wall and the commentator's voice intoning, "Broadmoor. A name with fear built into it". Dr Chandra Ghosh photographed well and was interviewed saying that men were in Special Hospitals for far more serious crimes than most of the women, men constituted far more of the mad axe category but women's crimes (termed index offences) were often trivial. It was thus wrong to put women into Broadmoor. I was staggered that Chandra was saying what I had campaigned about since my arrival fourteen years earlier. I had been shocked to find the girls on the Block, Lancs House, were largely epileptic and they needed caring for not humiliating with a harsh regime.

Memories of Jackie Hodge, I'd bought strawberries and cream for the ward for her twenty first birthday party. She would organize the ward, "Play canasta JC?". When she committed suicide I cried. Nejla, a pretty eighteen year old abandoned at London Airport by her husband who had flown her over from Cyprus and taken the next plane back. She had been taken to Long Grove at Epsom and, from there, dumped on Broadmoor. It was only a visiting nurse from Long Grove who told the staff what had happened. "Faggy faggy fuck fuck" was practically all Nejla could say in

English. "We can't send her back because of the political situation" said a Nursing Officer.

I had reached the point long ago when I left the replies to my letters of complaint unopened, there were now a bundle of them in the Stores, as I could see for myself that nothing was done. Yet here was the female wing psychiatrist saying openly what I knew to be a major malfunction in the mental health services and it left me wondering how much influence she had in dictating which patients were accepted by Broadmoor and which rejected. It also sunk in what my friend from Hereford had told me. Chandra was in trouble for having her husband in Holloway diverting those patients they thought should be in Broadmoor. Both were threatened with dismissal, the husband was transferred to Wormwood Scrubs, Chandra Ghosh to the male parole ward where she was obliged to organize the transfer of the male patients from whom she had endeavoured to protect vulnerable female patients. She ultimately left Broadmoor completely but that was later.

The film showed Annie who had been packed and ready to leave when an injunction was put on her; Marian P who had been out in the community for some years but the system would not let go and she was still required to attend tribunal hearings. When I arrived in Holloway in 1976 Marian had been on the point of leaving for Broadmoor, she had not been on a Section 43 (no contact with other prisoners), which was placed on me. Terry who I remembered removed my wet washing from the drier to put hers in, who's offence was so minor and who now worked as a plasterer. There were other tales of woe and injustice. To the commentator's voice saying, "Janet Cresswell has been in Broadmoor for fourteen years" a rather fey picture of me appeared on the screen, my voice slightly muffled from background noises in the Central Hall and there are captions of me saying, "In many ways I cannot hope too much otherwise it's disappointing. I just live day by day, week by week". Not for the first time I think my voice is rather like Princess Margaret launching a ship. Another interview with Ghosh saying of me, "It is difficult to decide why she was put in a psychiatric hospital or what treatment she could have been offered. As it is she has had none and been merely dumped in Broadmoor". Why, when she says this publicly on TV doesn't she write this in her statement for my tribunal?

Alvada greets me solefully. She too has viewed the film. Neither of us are in doubt that it will not impact in the way we both want despite its good intentions but it is surely a help in the right direction. Far more damaging are the grotesque accounts of our existence that appear regularly in some papers. There did appear to be a sense of right and wrong in those in positions of authority which those at the bottom subjected to it could rarely discern but sadly there is also a sense of possession, by authority, a refusal to let us go. We are both conscious of the patient with whom we were friendly who murdered her boyfriend, who was an alcoholic on the instruction of voices in the head. She had sailed through Broadmoor and was out in five years, the reason for this was being cured by Largactil. The victim was not a member of the medical profession. Neither Alvada nor I had even been given parole. She had learnt to fly on her uncle's crop sprayer so that she could be a ferry pilot back in the war, flying planes over to this country, I had wanted to join the WRNS and wear a pork pie hat but the war had ended before either of us fulfilled our ambitions. We were thus united by thwarted aspirations; cessation of hostilities can be a squasher of dreams as well as a liberation of others.

On Alvada's mind is her official Embassy visitor. It is custom for all foreign embassies to visit their nationals detained by their host country's judicial system. Zara, my downstairs neighbour when I lived in Hampstead, whose father and step-father had been in the diplomatic service, had once told me that accounts for detained foreigners were sent to the relative embassies and I had once commented to Alvada that it was cheaper for the USA to pay for her in Broadmoor than ship her back home; she had tossed this one off with a wave of the hand.

She tells me there is a new American Ambassador, traditionally this post is held by millionaires, Jo Kennedy had been one. This Ambassador is called Seitz, "a poor Jew" says Alvada. As a previous ambassador personally interviewed one of her official Embassy visitors, Alvada surmises that this one might do so too. It was therefore on the cards that Alvada might be mentioned to the new Ambassador. Here she went melancholy. "He'll support the Jewish lobby against me; he'll says I've got a hit list with George Pinker on it." She hasn't got a hit list, the authorities are paranoid. There is no Jewish lobby against her so she is paranoid and should be detained for perpetuity. One day sanity will emerge....What's new.....

MOVEMENT RATE FROM BROADMOOR'S FEMALE WING 1978 – 1992

(These figures would appear to reflect the relationship between politics of the day and the psychiatrist in charge. NB With a population of 120 a transfer rate of 6 women a year represents a 20-year stay. A leaflet of the 70's stated the average stay of a patient to be 4 years)

1978:	3 to old peoples homes.	**Total 3:120.**	Labour party in

1979:	1 repatriated to W. Indies after 4 years in Broadmoor. 1 to high security at Moss side. 4 to outside mental hospitals.	**Total 6:120**	Labour party defeated.

1980:	2 suicides (1 aged 22, epileptic, in B'moor 4 years for breaking windows in a B'moor for 20 years; committed suicide after demotion to the block for minor demeanour to create space on admission ward, the same reason as Liz Finch, who died in 1977) 2 to high security at Moss Side. 4 to """"Rampton. 2 to hostels (1 returned). 14 to outside mental hospitals.	**Total 24:120**	

1981:	2 to hostels. 1 to Scottish High Security at Carstairs. 13 to outside mental hospitals. 1 died (in 60's, natural causes).	**Total: 17**	Patient numbers reduced to 97 – 100, decreasing steadily to around 50 by 2000.

1982	1 went home (believed innocent of crime) 5 to other high security hospitals. 3 to outside mental hospitals (1 returned) 2 to hostels 1 died (mid 40's, from pneumonia).	**Total: 12**	

1983	9 to outside mental hospitals.	**Total: 9**	**MHA amended.**

1984	1 transferred to prison. 1 to high security at Moss Side. 9 to outside mental hospital (1 returned). 1 to hostel. 2 died (both natural causes)	Total: 14	
1985	2 transferred to prison. 8 to outside mental hospitals (2 returned). 1 suicide (early 30's).	Total: 11	
1986	9 to outside mental hospitals. 1 to hostel. 2 died (1 from an "internal blockage" – constipation. The other in 70's from natural causes.	Total: 12	
1987	5 to outside mental hospitals. 1 to high security at Rampton. 2 died (1 in 70's, natural causes. The 2nd in 60's of cancer which was not diagnosed until autopsy).	Total: 8	RMO ill, leaves and subsequently dies. Replaced with new RMO and registrar.
1988	12 to outside mental hospitals. 2 to high security at Rampton. 1 to hostel. 1 home (discharged	Total: 16	

from block to commit suicide within a few weeks).

1989   1 to prison.
18 to outside mental hospitals.
1 to hostel.
2 home.
1 died (aged 68, natural causes).

Total: 23

1990   4 died (1 aged 41 – coronary. 2nd aged 40 chocked on peanut butter sandwich. 2 suicides, 1 aged 65 after 40 years in Broadmoor, and 1 aged 24).
1 to high security at Moss Side.
6 to outside mental hospitals.
2 to hostel (1 returned but re-transferred).

Total: 13

1991   8 to regional secure units (RSI): 4 returned, 1 re-offended and commit suicide.
9 to outside mental hospitals.
3 to hostels.
1 transferred to prison.
3 home.
1 died.

Total: 25

RMO reprimanded for too many transfers and transferred to male side.

1992   5 to RSU's.   **Total: 8**
2 to outside mental hospitals.
1 home to re-offend and be sent to
prison.

APPENDIX - A USER'S REPORT ON PSYCHIATRIC SERVICES

Janet Cresswell is a patient at Broadmoor and had the initiative to conduct a survey helped by Patrick Woods, a Barnsley Community Care Worker.

Asylum felt this initiative required recognition and are pleased that it is possible for someone in a Special Hospital to be able to do it. It says something complimentary about both.

Janet was a secretary once working in the same office as Norman Lamont then an opposition MP. She was co-author of the play 'The One-sided Wall', a talking heads piece about a woman's psychiatric experiences. She says she lived in Hampstead where the ratio of psychiatrists per capita was the highest in Europe. She was married to an architect, has one daughter and two grand-children. She has been in Broadmoor for 16 years.

She had an article published in the Sunday Times colour supplement 'A Day in the Life of....' series. Whatever the reason for her incarceration we wish her well.

THE SURVEY

The survey was felt to be necessary as, despite there being no test for insanity, the UK has the highest mental illness rate in Western Europe (*85 people took part in this survey which was conducted in 1992).* This seemed to be at variance with benefits available. An overwhelming 76% of people say that psychiatric treatment did not cure them, 5% say there was nothing to cure. Further problems to the ones for which help was originally sought were experienced by over half the users. Despite this, contributors were reluctant to vote for the complete abolition of all mental health services. Whereas 38% users voted for the complete abolition of psychiatry, 46% wanted its continuation although many stated there should be more counseling and switching of funds from hospital to community based services. The suffering of many users under the heading medical treatment is an indictment of the medical profession.

1. USERS WERE ASKED WHEN THEY HAD FIRST RECEIVED PSYCHIATRIC TREAMENT.

The survey included several users who had first received psychiatric treatment as far back as 1945. Those committed at that time and the 1960's were the most vehement in their anti-psychiatry views and most adamant that their treatments had caused far more problems than cured.

2. USERS WERE ASKED TO STATE THE REASON FOR THEIR FIRST PSYCHIATRIC INVOLVEMENT.

Emotional/domestic insecurity - 49% (including, loneliness; immigration; adolescence; panic attacks etc)
Depression - 8% (including 3% post-natal depression and 2% suicide attempts)
Homelessness - 8%
Paranormal experiences - 3% (although 7% experienced these phenomena they had originally received treatment for other reasons, mainly insecurity)
Business worries/breakdown from work - 2%
Brain damage - 1%
Anxiety from physical illness -1%

Not suffering from insanity - 4% (Fear by others was attributed as reasons for committals/treatment)

OTHER, described as:

Hypermania – 6%
Withdrawal from problems – 6%
Schizophrenic symptoms – 6%
Parental problems – 6%
Victims of physical violence - 6%
Unstated - 12%

3. HAD USERS BEEN VOLUNTARY OR COMMITTED PATIENTS?

Committed under Mental Health Act - 34%
Voluntary - 42%
Both voluntary and committed - 12%
Day Centres - 2%
Unaware of legal status of hospitalization - 10%

There were several instances of multiple committals, generally under three months' duration with one of thirty years in a mental hospital stemming from adolescent problems and hospitalizations at the age of thirteen causing greater problems with educational setbacks. As 42% at some time had been voluntary patients (several had been cajoled into accepting treatment) it was felt that these would be less prone to antagonism at the psychiatric services than those who had been forcibly detained. This hypothesis was not borne out by the survey.

4. & 5. USERS WERE ASKED TO LIST THE TREATMENT THEY HAD REQUIRED AND RECEIVED.

Treatment required:

Sympathetic, (including rape and legal) counseling and common sense - 32% (rarely forthcoming)
Drugs (usually tranquillizers) - 29% (usually prescribed)
Psychotherapy and analysis - 10% (4% received some form)
Cure for insecurity and depression - 20% (all medicated)
Explanation for committal - 3% (no explanation given medicated)
Rest - 3%
ECT - 3% (27% had had ECT many of whom campaigned for its withdrawal)
Sex therapy - 2% (all medicated)
Love, Respect, Housing Benefit help, Referral to homosexual group, Art therapy - Change of diet, (food intolerance) - 8%. All medicated. Some art therapy.
Don't know - 3% (Figures add to over 100% as some stated more than one requirement)

Treatment Received:

Most people had been medicated and many complained of side effects, some long lasting. The practice of multi-medication (prescribing several different tranquillises simultaneously) was considered unfortunate and the reintroduction of lithium deprecated. Whereas tranquillisers were considered necessary in many instances, it was considered that drugs were frequently prescribed unnecessarily and for too long a period. Withdrawal of medications was sometimes too abrupt and should be handled more carefully. One user had been forced to take LSD in 1966 and another had received 50 "mild" induced insulin comas. These people, with those receiving ECT without anaesthetic suffered grossly out of proportion to the complaint originally sought to be relieved but medication of more recent years (including those by injection) is not always welcomed. One had undergone a leucotomy which today is out of fashion.

31% had received **group therapy.** Any benefit from this was dependent largely on the composition of the group. It is unusual for anyone to say very much as there is a natural reluctance to discuss personal problems in public, or for one person to take all the attention with fairly trivial matters. As a means of occupying time and providing a get-together, group therapy is considered relatively harmless.

Psychoanalysis, "know yourself", is felt to be therapeutic but too much introspection and continual reliving past events is regarded as retarding natural development.

ECT remains controversial, very few users asking for this but others are vehement that it should be outlawed.

Occupational therapy, including art, music and education, is welcomed.

Most people respond to a stable **routine** with three meals a day and a **good night's sleep** (not always easy without night medication in a locked ward) but if detained for too long a period, they become restless resulting in greater need for activity.

Case Conferences, whereby an absent user is discussed by a number of staff, is regarded, in many instances, as legalised slander.

The recent change in the law, whereby people can have sight of their medical records, has left several users in disbelief at the way they and their histories are recorded.

6. HAD THE TREATMENT CURED THE USER?

Not cured – 76%
Nothing to cure – 5%
Unsure – 7%
(Partly) stabilised – 5%

Cured – 10% (*see below)
Some insight into problems – 4%
Unwanted side effects of treatment – 50%

Note: Side effects commented on include: Addiction to tranquillisers, Cured of all hospitals, Cured of professionals, Hormonal upsets, Intense migraines, Less able to cope with problems, Loss of employment, Loss of home, Lowering of self-esteem and confidence, Memory loss, Mental stigma (resulting in further psychological and employment problems, Bans on emigration, Insurance difficulties, Pilferage of belongings, Resentment at authority for allowing psychiatric treatment, Side effects of medication (several very unpleasant), Tuned to alternative medicine, Turned to religion.

*The image that mental illness can be treated successfully with one hospitalisation of six weeks or so is an idyll but materialised rarely in the survey sheets. One user had been committed six times over a period of nine years before being put on depixol injections which were claimed to have cured 'psychotic symptoms'. Another had been cured "each time" (eight hospitalisations). As there are numerous instances of users relapsing on this same medication it was felt that a hospital routine, or relief from an environment, was perhaps the stabilising factor. Other successful cures were attributed to having security of home and well paid job to return to. One appeared to be a hospital worker who was more able, perhaps, to assess the help given. Thus the figure of 10% cure by conventional means is more likely to be around 2% in real terms.

7. FOR WHAT REASON DO USERS SEE A PSYCHIATRIST REGULARLY?

For helpful advice/support – 22%
Release conditions of court order – 10%
Attend day centre/psychotherapist/community work – 3%
Do not see a psychiatrist – 65%

Some people felt psychiatrists, as against not having enough knowledge, were too adept in sadistic ability. Several were adamant that they would never again consult any psychiatrist.

8. ASKED IF CURES COULD HAVE BEEN EFFECTED IF....

	Yes	No	Don't know
The psychiatrist had more time and staff	20%	41%	5%
The user was more responsive	18%	41%	4%
The psychiatrist had more knowledge	29%	42%	8%

Many stressed that there was either nothing to cure or that nothing could cure them. Others asked who could judge a cure.

9. USERS WERE ASKED IF THOSE WITH LOWER MENTAL CAPACITIES SHOULD BE DETAINED IN MENTAL HOSPITALS IN THE SAME MANNER AS CRIMINALS CONVICTED THROUGH THE COURTS TO MENTAL HOSPITALS:

Yes – 7%
No – 72%
Don't know – 21%
(Notes in 10 apply)

10. USERS WERE ASKED IFTHEY BELIEVED THE POLICY OF CHANNELLING PRISONERS FROM THE COURTS TO MENTAL HOSPITALS WAS UPSETTING TO GENUINELY CONFUSED PATIENTS.

Yes – 77%
No – 10%
Don't know – 13%

Note: This policy gained momentum in the 1970's. Whilst it can be argued that all crime is insane, this is academic and in real terms there is a great difference between a law-abiding person experiencing a nervous breakdown and one on a vandalism spree. Several users were very adamant, scoring heavily under their answers and writing comments, that some people had been very upset indeed to find themselves treated in the same fashion as rapists and shoplifters.

The policy of relieving prison overcrowding by sending prisoners to mental hospitals may have been convenient to the Home Office but has caused untold damage to the genuinely mentally ill. the upsurge of this policy coincided with the repeal of the death sentence which required psychiatric opinion to decide on the insanity loophole and for some while it appeared as though psychiatric intervention in the legal system was under threat. Thus the search for their own identity by psychiatrists is seen as conflicting with the needs of society.

11. USERS WERE ASKED IF THEY FELT THAT MONIES SPENT ON PSYCHIATRIC SERVICES COULD BE BETTER UTILISED IF CHANNELLED INTO IMPROVED HOUSING, CHILD MINDING SERVICES, SPORT AND ENTERTAINMENT FACILITIES IN THE COMMUNITY:

Yes – 54%
No – 40%
Don't know – 6%
One user felt all entertainment and sport waste of public resource, others stressed the need for security of tenure and housing for everybody. Several stressed the need for counselling which the State did not adequately provide. Counselling was more likely to be met by user services on a voluntary basis.

12. USERS WERE ASKED THEY HAD COMPLAINED OF PSYCHIATRIC TREATMENT, TO WHOM AND WITH WHAT RESULT:

Only 4% of the 44% who complained had received any satisfactory response to their complaints. **Complaints** to official organisations such as the Health Ombudsman, DHS, General Medical Council, British Medical Association and so on produced placatory, unsatisfactory responses. A Community Health Council showed concern and intervened to some extent. MIND were considered helpful. Appeals to second-opinion psychiatrists about medication (allowed by law) were not considered helpful. One committal order was lifted before the appeal was heard. One received an out of court settlement for a prescribed drugs overdose and appeared the only one to receive compensation. Other complaints are still pending.

Complaints covered a wide range of issues – poor hygiene in hospitals, food shortages, medication, treatment generally (including medication and by staff) noise problems. It is interesting that so much time and effort is taken by the authorities to muffle complaints and it is noticeable that the system has been amended, the 1983 MHA Amendments Act contributing to this. Mental

Health Commissioners, recruited from within the mental health system, pay regular visits to all mental hospitals to hear complaints but these received no mention in the survey, presumably as most contributors to it were now in the community.

In several instances users felt that, as a result of complaining, their treatment worsened, and this indicated a paranoia in locally based staff who could not tolerate criticism. Many users were too frightened to complain. Concern was expressed at the manner in which claims against drug companies were manipulated. In one case it was stated that 17,000 legal aid forms had been distributed entailing the diversion of nearly £7M of public monies to be paid to "authorised" psychiatrists for them to advise claimants of the invalidity of their claim. Presumably the legal profession were also beneficiaries from this exercise.

15. USERS WERE ASKED FOR ANY OTHER COMMENTS:

Several users commented that psychiatric training was too clinical, thus rendering the psychiatrist less able to understand or tolerate emotions and feelings in others. It was thought that psychologists might be more suitable for counselling. Several complained of coercement to take medication, being threatened with instant discharge or renewal of section, whichever was convenient. Overall, it was felt that users should be allowed to refuse treatment without threats of alternative pressure and regardless of the legal status of the treatment. Fear of medication or other treatment prevented some people from mentioning such matters as paranormal experiences (extra sensory perception ESP) not regarded as insanity by many. There is now a movement towards "legalising" these experiences.

The Mental Health Act is too easily manipulated to hold people on doubts, suspicions and fears, termed "opinion" rather than evidence of mental disorder which is not based on hard facts. On the other hand there are several instances of people being discharged from hospitals and wandering the streets to be picked up by the police showing a lack of responsibility by the hospital authorities. "How can a person on invalidity pay live a normal life?" asked one. Several users objected to being told they needed their medication for ever and having to pay for subscriptions. The need for housing for everybody and cheaper entertainment and sports facilities was underlined. Supportive housing schemes, 24-hour crisis centres and any other non-hospital refuge in times of crisis were thought preferable to hospitalisation. People should be encouraged to cope for themselves but, if they do, their problems are more likely to be ignored. Thus psychiatry erodes self-help whilst doing little or nothing to minimise th4 problems. Several people felt they gave more support to other patients than offered by staff. Education was needed for the general public to be allowed to express feelings openly without giving offence. More friendliness in the community was required.

SUMMARY

At medical school, students are informed that there are known cures for twenty-six diseases – mental illness is not one of them and treatments have frequently exceeded in insanity the insanity sought to cure. Refusal to admit limitations waste inestimable sums of public monies and adds to the suffering emanating from unhelpful treatment. Those who are able to enter into agreement with their psychiatrists that there is nothing he can do, fare better than those who expect cures. With so much expertise evident at diverting and stifling complaints, it is indeed surprising that more cures are not forthcoming. The insensitivity of some consultants is highlighted by the man who was tortured with electric shock treatment by foreign secret police to be given ECT for depression in this country.

Despite being told to take drugs indefinitely, many users stopped taking medication and benefited accordingly; it does seem that medication generally is prescribed for too long a period.

Social workers, although forming a significant part of the mental health empire, received no mention by users; the legal profession would appear to be the beneficiaries from the system, particularly with regard to tribunals.

Over a third of psychiatric users would like to see psychiatry abolished completely, believing that nothing is better than something that is harmful. For 48% of users to vote for the continuation of psychiatric services, despite results, shows an optimism over experience and this attitude is supported by 18% who were willing to believe that it was their lack of response to the treatment and nothing else that provided no relief. Many stated that they had joined self-help groups whose aim is to improve services. A majority of 54.40% of users were in favour of monies at present being spent on psychiatric services being switched into the community in the form of crisis and counselling centres, improved housing, child minding, sport and entertainment. Most of these facilities being outside the financial reach of many users. It is significant that there appears a marked difference in the results of hospitalised treatment between those with home and jobs to return to, which substantiates the need for better housing and more, and less costly, occupational facilities in the community. As the diagnosis of mental illness relies so much on opinion, personal prejudice can be a factor of treatment and detention which is undesirable. Unless the law is broken, detention and treatment should be on a voluntary basis. those who break the law should receive definite sentences. Not least is the hope that if the community could be encouraged to be more friendly, allowing old ladies out at night without fear of attack, the problem of mental illness, from emotional and depressive disorders, would be reduced enormously.

This survey originally appeared in *Asylum* 22, Spring 1993.

Printed in the United Kingdom
by Lightning Source UK Ltd.
119134UK00001B/23